SURVIVING
PROSTATE
CANCER
WITHOUT
SURGERY:
THE NEW GOLD
STANDARD
TREATMENT
THAT CAN SAVE
YOUR LIFE AND
LIFESTYLE

SURVIVING PROSTATE CANCER WITHOUT SURGERY:

THE NEW GOLD STANDARD TREATMENT THAT CAN SAVE YOUR LIFE AND LIFESTYLE

MICHAEL J. DATTOLI, MD

JENNIFER CASH, ARNP, MS, OCN

DON KALTENBACH, PROSTATE CANCER SURVIVOR

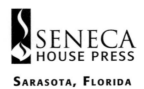

SENECA
HOUSE PRESS

SARASOTA, FLORIDA

Published by Seneca House Press, Sarasota, Florida.

ISBN: 0964008882

Library of Congress Control Number: 2004114137

For information on distributor to the trade in the United States, contact:
Seneca House Press / Dattoli Cancer Foundation, 2803 Fruitville Road, Sarasota, FL 34237 (800-915-1001)

Book design and composition by Design Corps, Batavia, IL

Printed by Marrakesh Express, Tarpon Springs, Florida

DEDICATION

This book is dedicated to all those whose lives have been touched by prostate cancer, and to the patients and their families whom we are privileged to serve and educate as cancer care providers.

MEDICAL DISCLAIMER

This book is intended as a supplement but not as a substitute for the medical advice of a physician. It is imperative that you consult a qualified healthcare professional with regard to all matters relating to your health and particular situation. Neither the publisher nor the authors bear responsibility for any consequences due to the reader's decision to use any particular treatment, medication, dietary supplement or other healthcare practices discussed in this book.

ACKNOWLEDGMENTS

We are grateful to a number of people who have contributed to this book in a variety of ways. Our thanks to Greg Lawrence, for his editorial efforts and enthusiastic devotion to the project and to Dawn Horowitz, Ginya Carnahan, and Bets Burrell for their ongoing support and organizational efforts.

We deeply appreciate all the wonderful patients and family members who have contacted the Dattoli Cancer Foundation for counseling and guidance and in turn have given us their support and encouragement. It is your commitment and spirit in confronting this disease that inspires us all!

CONTENTS

Part One—The Non-Surgical Approach to Diagnosis and Treatment

by Michael Dattoli, M.D.

Part Two—The Patient's Point of View

by Don Kaltenbach

Part Three—Post-treatment Care and Lifestyle Changes

by Jennifer Cash, ARNP, MS, OCN®

Appendices

INTRODUCTION
BY DON KALTENBACH

I f you are reading this book, chances are that you or someone in your life has been diagnosed with prostate cancer. The first thing you should know is that the situation is not as dire as it might seem. There is no reason for panic. Because this form of cancer is usually slow-growing, you have time to learn about the disease and fully assess your treatment options. The good news is that there are a number of effective treatments available and most men can now survive prostate cancer without having to undergo major surgery.

As a prostate cancer survivor and as director of one of the country's premier institutions for prostate cancer research and treatment, I encourage patients to work closely with their doctors and to learn all they can before deciding on treatment. Since I was treated in 1990, dramatic progress has been made in diagnosing and curing the disease. In fact, this field of medicine has changed so rapidly that most books on the subject, even those published within the past few years, are woefully out of date. This is partly due to the fact that most books about prostate cancer have been written primarily from a surgical perspective. By contrast, the authors of this book are all involved with state-of-the-art radiation therapy, which according to the most recent Medicare data, has now surpassed surgery as the mainstream treatment of choice (see Figure 1).

Why the trend away from surgery? The PSA blood test has transformed the entire field of prostate cancer research by enabling doctors not only to diagnose the disease earlier, but to more accurately determine the cure rates for each type of treatment. Back in the 1990's, most men with early stage prostate cancer were advised to have their prostates removed by the surgical procedure known as radical prostatectomy. At that time, surgery was considered the "gold standard" treatment. But more recently, the majority of patients have been choosing to avoid the knife, opting instead for sophisticated forms of radiation therapy, such as radioactive seed implants or brachytherapy (pronounced brăk-ē-therapy) and Intensity Modulated Radiation Therapy (IMRT). These combined therapies are proving superior both in terms of cure rates and preserving quality of life. Over the past decade, I have had a special interest in seeding because this was the form of treatment that I chose for myself when it was still investigational, before ten and twelve year studies demonstrated its advantages over surgery.

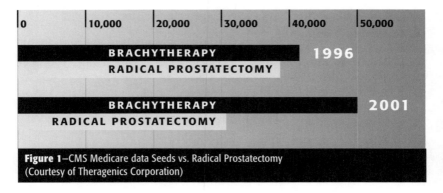

Figure 1—CMS Medicare data Seeds vs. Radical Prostatectomy (Courtesy of Theragenics Corporation)

The purpose of this book is to provide you with the most reliable and up to date information to guide you from diagnosis to recovery. Before making any decisions about treatment, you should fully investigate the pros and cons of each form of therapy—the likelihood of cure and the risk of long-term side effects that may alter your quality of life. Taking into account your age, your overall health, and the extent of the cancer, you will want to find a balance between treatment effectiveness and side effects—a balance with which you are comfortable, that you can live with both before and after treatment. Regardless of which type of therapy you may decide is right for you, knowing what to expect is one of the keys to fighting this disease.

You should also be aware from the outset that doctors continue to disagree about which treatment is best and whether treatment is necessary. There are many conflicting viewpoints and many misconceptions that find their way into the media. Therefore, it is often wise to obtain second opinions from one or more specialists within the field. Like all of us, doctors have biases. They tend to recommend what they know how to do: urologists tend to recommend surgery; radiation oncologists tend to favor radiation. If you have received advice from a surgeon, then you should do yourself the favor of seeking an opinion from a radiation oncologist, and vice versa. Each of these specialists will be better able to explain how and why he does what he does. The data and quality of life issues, however, will ultimately speak for themselves as you do your own research and compare the results for each type of treatment for which you may be eligible. This book will emphasize radiation as the newly emergent gold standard therapy and give you additional guidance as you make your way through what can sometimes seem like a bewildering maze of options.

Why Get a Second Opinion?

Deciding which treatment is right for you is like shopping for a car. You go to a Ford dealer, you go to a Chevrolet dealer, and you go to a Chrysler dealer. Each dealer has a different product and approach. So it is with doctors. When you go to a surgeon to discuss treatment options, he is likely to have a greater comfort level with surgery because of his training and practice. Likewise, a radiation oncologist is likely to be more comfortable with radiation. Find out from each type of doctor exactly what he does and how he does it.

What This Book Offers

Treating prostate cancer successfully requires the combined efforts of doctors, nurses and patients, and each of those three essential points of view will be offered in the pages ahead. The authors are experienced healthcare professionals associated with the Dattoli Cancer Center & Brachytherapy Research Institute in Sarasota, Florida. The three of us, each working from a different vantage, are dedicated to the treatment of prostate cancer. Dr. Michael Dattoli is one of the country's leading radiation oncologists and brachytherapists, with numerous published studies to his credit and one of the highest cure rates in the field. In the first part of the book, he will explain his cutting edge approach to diagnosis and treatment, offering the same practical advice he gives to his own patients. Jennifer Cash is an Advanced Registered Nurse Practitioner (ARNP) who specializes in the care of prostate cancer patients who receive radiation therapy. In the second part of the book, she will explain in common sense terms how you can prepare yourself for treatment and what you can anticipate after being treated.

As a former patient, I can tell you that in addition to the physical side of the disease, prostate cancer is an emotional journey. The prospect of having to cope with any life-threatening disease can be harrowing. It is not just the medical tests and wading through statistics. Prostate cancer affects us on the deepest gut levels. Developing a positive mental outlook can make a world of difference in the long run. While every individual case is unique, there are challenging aspects of this disease that all of us experience. I will discuss these areas in the third part of this book, from the vantage of my having already made the passage and lived through what you are likely to be going through.

As a lawyer, I also want to make you aware of your rights as a patient. Our shared goal with this book is to help you make *informed decisions* about your treatment. Don't delegate that decision to someone else. After all, it's your body and your health that are at stake. As you gather information, always consider the source and use your own judgment about your needs. *You will know best what is right for you.* Don't be afraid to voice your concerns to your doctor and don't hesitate to ask questions—you have every right to know the answers and to expect a standard of care with which you are satisfied. It is my dearest hope that those of us who have made this journey before you can help you find your way more readily, that the path will be easier for you, and your destination all the more sure.

PART ONE

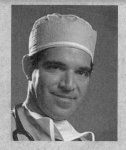

BY MICHAEL DATTOLI, M.D

THE NON-SURGICAL APPROACH TO DIAGNOSIS AND TREATMENT

The entire field of prostate cancer diagnosis and treatment has undergone a revolution during the past few decades, in part brought about by widespread screening with the PSA blood test, which has allowed for earlier diagnosis of the disease. We have also seen dramatic technological progress in each of the medical specialties that are involved in the field. All of these changes have improved the prognosis for most patients regardless of their age and the stage of their cancers.

Recent advances in the delivery of high energy photons, ultrasound imaging, and computerized treatment planning have essentially turned the tide against what was previously thought to be a disease most effectively treated by means of radical surgery. At this time, an overview of prostate cancer care and treatment from a non-surgical perspective, as presented in this book, is crucial for every patient wishing to receive the highest standard of care. The discussion that follows is intended to provide the latest data and essential knowledge to prepare patients to make fully informed decisions about their treatment options with their doctors.

CHAPTER ONE

THE BASICS OF PROSTATE CANCER

What is prostate cancer?

Prostate cancer (PCa) is the most commonly diagnosed cancer in men. Since the advent of screening with the PSA blood test in the late 1980's, prostate cancer has been diagnosed more frequently, reaching epidemic proportions during the last decade. It is second only to lung cancer as a leading cause of cancer death in the male population. That grim statistic, however, is likely to change as the disease is increasingly diagnosed earlier when it is more treatable.

Where is the Prostate Gland Located and what is its Function?

The prostate is a walnut-size gland located at the bottom of the pelvis, just beneath the bladder and in front of the rectum (see Figure 2). Found only in men, the prostate gland surrounds an inch-long segment of the urethra, the channel through which urine exits the bladder and passes out of the body. The primary function of the prostate is to produce some of the seminal fluid, which flows into the urethra at the time of orgasm. The fluid allows for nourishment and transport of the sperm at ejaculation. The seminal vesicles are two sac-like structures that are attached to the back of the prostate and produce additional seminal fluid that passes through the gland.

The prostate gland contains many hundreds of tiny passageways lined with cells that produce seminal fluid. Normally, these lining cells reproduce slowly, at about the same rate that cells die. But with cancer, some of these cells become abnormal and reproduce at an uncontrollable rate. Although several other cell types are found in the prostate, more than 99% of prostate cancers develop from the glandular cells. The medical term for cancer that starts in glandular cells like these is *adenocarcinoma.* Over time, the build-up of cancerous cells in the gland produces a lump or "tumor." Not all tumors are cancerous. Benign tumors can be caused by infections, bruising and other nonmalignant medical conditions.

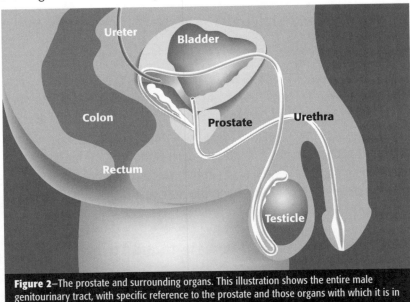

Figure 2–The prostate and surrounding organs. This illustration shows the entire male genitourinary tract, with specific reference to the prostate and those organs with which it is in close relationship.

It should be noted that prostate cancer is not contagious. Nor can it be sexually transmitted. Because prostate cancer grows so slowly, it often causes no symptoms in the early stages. When symptoms do occur, they usually take the form of difficult or frequent urination, a slow or weak urine stream and/or urination during the night (nocturia). These same symptoms, however, are more often caused by an overgrowth of normal prostate tissue that commonly occurs with aging. This non-cancerous condition is known as benign prostatic hypertrophy, or BPH (See Figure 3).

Although many men with BPH never experience serious problems due to the condition, with sufficient time, symptoms will begin to manifest. As

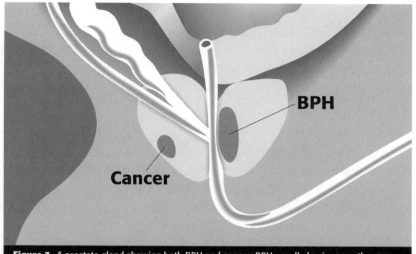

Figure 3—A prostate gland showing both BPH and cancer. BPH usually begins near the core, while prostate cancer more often arises near the boundary of the gland.

the prostate gland enlarges, BPH tissue may constrict the urethra. There are a variety of medications that can be used to treat the symptoms of BPH. These include alpha blockers like Hytrin® and Flomax®, and other agents such as Proscar® and Avodart®. With advanced BPH, surgery may be necessary. The most common surgical approach to BPH is called a *transurethral resection of the prostate* (TURP). For this procedure, the surgeon uses an instrument called a resectoscope to remove excess BPH tissue. In some cases when the prostate gland is very enlarged due to BPH, an open surgical procedure known as a *simple prostatectomy* may be performed. Other treatment methods take advantage of the fact that heat (thermopathy) eradicates benign cells (e.g. the indigo laser or the Targis™ microwave system).

How Common is Prostate Cancer?

According to the American Cancer Society, more than 230,000 men will be diagnosed with prostate cancer in 2004, and approximately 29,900 men will die from the disease. 1 out of 6 men will be diagnosed with prostate cancer during his lifetime, but only 1 out of 32 men will die from it. Prostate cancer becomes more prevalent with age. More than 70% of all prostate cancer cases are diagnosed in patients over age 65. Because the

U.S. has a rapidly aging population, the problem is on the rise. Many physicians are also seeing a growing number of younger patients, from 30 to 65. Whether this is due to earlier screening and detection or disease migration to younger individuals is currently unknown.

Symptoms of Prostate Cancer

✔ Blood in urine (hematuria).*
✔ Pain or difficulty urinating.*
✔ Increased frequency of urination, often at night (nocturia).*
✔ Hesitant or intermittent urinary flow.*
✔ Inability to urinate
✔ Pain or discomfort in area of prostate
✔ Unusual and unexplained weight loss.
✔ Continual pain in bones of lower back, hips or pelvis.

Note: Those symptoms marked with an * may be due to benign conditions of the prostate, entirely unrelated to prostate cancer.

What Causes Prostate Cancer?

The exact causes of prostate cancer are unknown, but a combination of genetic and environmental factors, including certain aspects of the lifestyle in western countries, probably contributes to the progression of the disease. Researchers have identified several inherited genes that appear to increase the risk of prostate cancer. We know that at least 10% of prostate cancers are inherited directly from parents, while most prostate cancers appear to be acquired because of the way we live and what we are exposed to in the environment. These non-genetic factors may include diet, smoking, industrial pollution, excessive alcohol consumption, stress, and so forth.

Autopsy studies have shown that in men over the age of 30, about a third will have microscopic prostate cancer regardless of their geographical location. Yet there is a gross discrepancy between the high rate of clinical prostate cancer in the U.S. and Western Europe compared to that in Asian countries like Japan. So it would seem there is something that keeps the microscopic cancer localized in Asian men, while the cancer is not contained in western men. This finding is strengthened by studies showing that for Asian men who migrate to the U.S., the incidence of clinical prostate cancer increases up to seven times in one generation. One factor that researchers believe may account for the geographical discrepancy with prostate cancer is diet, especially, the higher intake of saturated fat and red meat in the U.S. and Western Europe compared to Asia.

Who is Most at Risk for Prostate Cancer?

Age, race and family history are the most important risk factors for prostate cancer. Those men who are most at risk are those with a positive family history, Caucasians 50 years of age or older, and African American males over 40 years of age. Prostate cancer occurs almost 70% more often in African-American men than it does in white American men, and African Americans have the highest prostate cancer mortality rates of any ethnic group.

Studies also indicate that men with a family history of the disease are two or three times more likely to get prostate cancer. The likelihood that a man will inherit the disease increases if 1) two generations of his family have had prostate cancer, 2) two or more immediate relatives have had prostate cancer (brothers and/or father), and 3) one or more relatives are diagnosed before the age of 55. Men who have a strong family history of prostate cancer should begin yearly monitoring (with the PSA test and digital rectal exam) as early as age 35.

What Types of Doctors Treat Prostate Cancer?

The treatment of prostate cancer is divided between several medical specialties: urologists (surgeons), radiation oncologists, and medical oncologists. Urologists are doctors who spend one year after medical school studying general surgery, and three additional years studying surgical treatment of the sexual organs and urinary tract. Radiation oncologists are doctors who spend one to three years after medical school studying general medicine and four additional years studying the use of radiation for treating all types of cancer. Medical oncologists spend three years after medical school studying internal medicine and two additional years studying the use of chemotherapy, and to a lesser degree studying hormonal therapies.

In many cases, the specialties overlap. Urologists sometimes perform radioactive seed implants, but require assistance from a qualified radiation oncologist in order to treat with radiation. Both urologists and radiation oncologists often prescribe hormonal therapy, as do medical oncologists. Most newly diagnosed patients are first referred to a urologist, and are often encouraged to have surgical treatment before they have had the opportunity to fully assess their other options. For this reason, patients are well advised not to rush into any form of treatment, to do their own research and obtain second opinions from the other specialties.

Why is the Treatment of Prostate Cancer so Controversial?

Part of the reason this field is controversial is due to the fact that regardless of which treatment is used, patients have a reasonable, short-term, disease-free prognosis, which is unlike most other cancers. This is true even for prostate cancer patients who undergo the more esoteric or investigational therapies. Even patients who choose not to be treated are most likely not going to die in the short term. In addition, when a primary therapy like radiation or surgery fails, there are other treatments like hormonal therapy or other systemic medications to fall back on. This is a different kind of situation than you find with most other diseases.

With other cancers, you're really put in a position where your back is against the wall and you're fighting for your life. As a doctor, you're in fifteenth round, and you have to knock this cancer out, or that's it for your patient. With prostate cancer, we have a variety of specialties, all of which offer treatments that can potentially knock the cancer out at least for a while. In this situation, each type of specialist can argue that the specialty he has been trained in and practices offers the best therapy.

In order for you as a patient to find your way through these conflicting viewpoints, a careful evaluation of the latest data on cure rates and quality of life is essential to consider along with the specifics of your case and your individual needs. This is especially important since despite the relatively slow growth of most prostate cancers, relapse may follow a slow, painful course. Many doctors believe that progressive prostate cancer is the worst type of cancer because it kills you slowly!

The argument over which type of treatment is best continues because there are no prospective randomized trials that would definitively compare the various specialties and the different treatments they offer. However, what we can do is rigorously compare the results obtained by the premier treatment centers for each specialty and each type of treatment. That type of comparison is available to both doctors and patients and probably explains why the trend is away from surgery, with an increasing number of patients choosing one or more forms radiation therapy.

How Do You Find the Doctor Who is Right For You?

A number of criteria can be used to help you evaluate a doctor's merit. A doctor with staff privileges at one or more hospitals will have usually demonstrated the necessary proficiency in his field to earn the respect of his or her colleagues. Review-committee membership at a respected medical institution also indicates a doctor's reputation among peers. A doctor whose practice is hospital-based or part of a group practice may be preferred, since any reputable hospital or group practice will require their physicians to undergo peer review sufficient to ensure quality care.

It is advisable to find a doctor who treats a large number of prostate cancer patients, and is therefore more familiar with the kind of care they require. Board certification will indicate that a doctor has been thoroughly examined although it cannot guarantee his competence. Certification in a specialty, especially oncology, or possession of a board fellowship are further indications of distinction. It is possible to check the credentials of a doctor with the Directory of Medical Specialists or the American Medical Directory, a copy of which can usually be found in the reference room of your local library. You might also ask a doctor for his or her curriculum vitae.

Any of these criteria will improve your chances of finding a capable physician. You might start as many patients do with a referral from a local, trusted doctor who is familiar with the reputable and respected physicians in your area. Keep in mind, however, that most general practitioners typically know very little about prostate cancer, and therefore, they usually refer prostate cancer patients to a urologist, who is likely to recommend surgical treatment rather than one of the non-surgical options.

A good physician will explain your condition in detail, taking the time to answer all of your questions and correcting any misconceptions you may have. It is your right to receive a complete description of all your options, and their advantages and disadvantages. This is vital information if you are to have a sense of control over what is happening to you. If the doctor fails to disclose this information, or does not encourage you to choose for yourself which treatment you wish to receive, find another doctor.

Throughout the period of your treatment, the physician should continue to keep you fully informed of the nature and rationale behind any tests or procedures recommended to you. Clear and concise written materials that explain the basic facts of prostate cancer, its symptoms and all of your treatment options, should also be made available to you.

A doctor who communicates concern for the patient as an individual can ease the treatment process. A physician who cares is more likely to inspire trust in his patients and help to allay their fears. But a doctor who sees each patient only as another medical condition to treat will most likely leave his patients feeling alienated, confused and anxious. Ultimately, such a doctor will impede the progress of those under his care.

In the final analysis, you need to have a comfort level with your doctor that enables to you answer the following questions affirmatively. Do you trust and have confidence in your doctor? Does he put you at ease? Are you able to talk with your doctor in a relaxed manner?

A physician may be completely suited for treating some patients and unsuited for treating others. It may be nothing more than a matter of incompatible personalities. But you will be making critical decisions with this doctor, and undergoing a treatment process that can be difficult and extend for months or even years. Is the physician only interested in treating you, or will he follow you after treatment annually or biannually? You will need a doctor you can depend on when the going gets tough. If for any reason you do not feel comfortable with your physician, you should carefully consider whether it is in your interests to find care elsewhere.

When Should Prostate Cancer not be Treated?

Studies have shown that with early stage prostate cancer patients who are not treated, the risk of dying from the disease is very low for the first 10 years after diagnosis. Therefore, in the past, it was argued that prostate cancer patients with a life expectancy of less than 10 years should not be treated, because they were more likely to die from some other cause. With life expectancy increasing for the population as a whole, there are actually fewer and fewer cases of prostate cancer these days that do not call for some form of treatment, and the relatively non-invasive therapies such as brachytherapy and/or IMRT are often appropriate for older men who are otherwise in good health.

According to the most recent actuarial data, a 60-year-old man has a life expectancy of 20 years or more. He should therefore pursue some form of treatment because he will probably live long enough to die from his prostate cancer if it isn't treated. An 80-year-old man now has a life expectancy of 9.1 years. In the case of an 80-year-old whose general health is good and who has no other serious health conditions, he too stands a good chance of living beyond 10 years and would also be wise to consider treatment. For men over 80, treatment should be determined on a case by case basis since their life expectancy begins to fall significantly below 10 years. Nonetheless, your health should be viewed as more important than age per se, since an 84 year old may actually be healthier than his 54 year old counterpart, who consumes excessive alcohol (ETOH abuse), smokes cigarettes, etc.

What is "Watchful Waiting" and when is it Recommended?

Watchful waiting is an option for some early stage prostate cancer patients who want to try to preserve their quality of life by avoiding aggressive treatment for their cancer at least temporarily. These men may be advised to wait and monitor the progression of their cancer with periodic laboratory tests and physical examinations. Although I inform my patients of this option, I'm generally opposed to it for most men, because I don't see much merit to the idea of waiting as cancer progresses and becomes less treatable. Nor do I see much data to support this approach. The exceptions are those patients regardless of age who have a life expectancy less than ten years because of some other medical condition, such as heart disease or another form of cancer that is likely to be a cause of death before prostate cancer. For these men, watchful waiting is a more realistic option.

Advocates of watchful waiting often correctly point out that the term is misleading and should not imply passive waiting or doing nothing. A more active program of surveillance (sometimes called "expectant management") is intended and may include a diet and fitness regimen undertaken in consultation with a doctor and tailored to the patient's condition. The process of waiting to see if the cancer progresses is bound to cause prolonged periods of anxiety for many men; and therefore, a strong sense of commitment and mental stamina are demanded of those who choose to wait rather than be treated.

Early proponents of watchful waiting based their argument on Swedish data, which received a great deal of publicity in the early 1990's. The Swedish researchers argued that there was no survival benefit for patients treated versus patients who were not treated. But if we look closely at those studies, it turns out that the patients were not just undergoing watchful waiting, because when the disease started to progress in men who had not been treated, they were subjected to endocrine therapies such as hormonal therapy or orchiectomy (castration). Therefore, the Swedish data did not provide an accurate picture of watchful waiting. As discussed in the next chapter, the survival benefits of treating prostate cancer have not yet been conclusively demonstrated, but researchers have compiled enough data to establish the long term cure rates for each type of treatment.

CHAPTER TWO

THE DIAGNOSTIC TESTS FOR PROSTATE CANCER

What is the Digital Rectal Exam (DRE)?

The digital rectal exam is the simplest way to detect physical abnormalities in the prostate gland that may suggest the presence of cancer. The DRE is also used to estimate the volume of the prostate and the extent of the cancer. The test is part of the physician's *work-up,* which involves a series of laboratory and radiographic tests that are used to determine how advanced the cancer is. The results of these tests will be evaluated to determine the *clinical stage* of the cancer, and they are also used to decide which type of treatment is most appropriate for your particular cancer.

To perform the rectal exam, the doctor feels the gland by placing a lubricated, gloved finger inside the rectum against the prostate (see Figure 4). When done properly, the test is not as discomforting as it might sound. Most cancers are located in the back of the prostate, and some of these cancers that have grown at the edge of the gland can be felt as a lump or hard nodule. Depending on the size, shape and location of the lump, it is sometimes possible to determine with a DRE if the cancer has spread beyond the prostate capsule. With the DRE, the doctor is able to evaluate the major portions of the gland's anatomy: the right and lefts sides or *lobes;* the upper portion or *base* of the gland; the middle portion of the gland; and lower portion or *apex.*

Unfortunately, the DRE is often not accurate. Many prostate cancers do not protrude against the back of the gland; they are not palpable and cannot be detected with the DRE. A tumor at the front of the prostate cannot

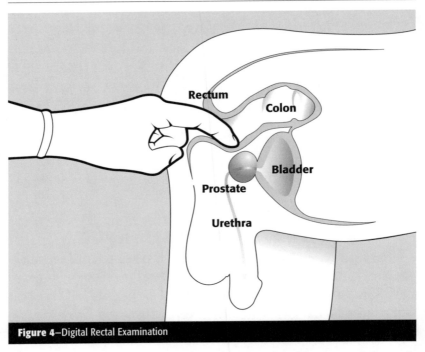

Figure 4–Digital Rectal Examination

be felt through the rectum. In addition, the test is subjective and depends on the skill of the doctor, providing at best only an estimate of the extent of disease. Many surgical studies have shown that more than 50% of cancers that appear to be confined to the gland will later be found to have spread beyond the prostate capsule. Once a tumor is palpable, there are more than a billion cancer cells.

What is the PSA test?

The PSA test was developed during the late 1970's by research scientists at Roswell Park Memorial Hospital in Buffalo, New York. The PSA is a blood test measures the amount of *prostate specific antigen* (PSA) present in the body. Produced almost exclusively by the prostate gland, PSA is an enzyme, typically present in only minute quantities, secreted into the bloodstream from blood vessels inside the prostate.

PSA secretions originate from cells in the lining of the prostate gland. The function of PSA appears to be liquefying the gelatinous semen and sustaining the viability of the sperm after ejaculation. When prostate cancer is present, additional PSA is usually produced. This extra PSA can be detected and measured in the blood through a simple laboratory test, which can be ordered by any primary-care physician. Test results are usually available in 1-3 days.

Because cancerous cells readily leak PSA into the surrounding body tissue, an elevated PSA is a possible indicator of the presence of prostate cancer. However, other conditions can also cause an elevated PSA. The most common is the enlargement of the prostate gland that occurs with BPH. Infections and traumas such as a biopsy or even an overly vigorous digital rectal exam can sometimes increase PSA levels. Ejaculation (orgasm) can elevate PSA for as long as 48 hours.

As a diagnostic tool, the PSA test has its limitations, and is usually combined with the DRE. Some men with seemingly normal PSA values turn out to have prostate cancer that may be detected with the DRE or by some other means. Though the PSA test is far from perfect as an indicator of cancer, in 1992 the American Cancer Society endorsed the idea of PSA/DRE screening for all men over age 50, and for those over 40 who are considered at higher risk (such as Afro-American males and those men with a family history of prostate cancer).

How Are PSA Results Reported?

Standard PSA test results are reported in nanograms per milliliter (ng/ml), with a normal range of approximately 0-4 ng/ml. For the sake of simplicity, the units of measure will not be included in the remainder of this book when discussing PSA values. The normal range of PSA values must be adjusted slightly to account for differences in age and race (see box below). As men get older, the normal PSA range slowly increases. This normal range is generally lower for White males than for Asians and Afro-Americans.

Regardless of age and race factors, PSA levels greater than 10 are most often an accurate indicator of cancer. As many as 80 percent of men with this high a PSA reading (and a positive digital rectal exam) have been shown to have prostate cancer. Approximately 25 percent of those patients with a PSA between 4 and 10 turn out to have cancer. The accuracy of the PSA test is significantly improved when it is combined with the digital rectal exam. The PSA can detect twice as many cancers as the DRE alone;

PSA–Typical ("Normal") range According to Age and Race

AGE	WHITE	ASIAN	AFRO-AMERICAN
40–49	0–2.5	0–2.0	0–2.0
50–59	0–3.5	0–3.0	0–2.0
60–69	0–4.5	0–4.0	0–4.5
70–79	0–6.5	0–5.0	0–5.5

however, the DRE spots some cancers that may be missed by the PSA.

It should be stressed that the PSA test is not conclusive by itself in diagnosing prostate cancer. No treatment decision should ever be made on the basis of the PSA value by itself; however, an elevated PSA reading may suggest the need for further laboratory tests. A biopsy of the prostate gland is always necessary to confirm the presence of cancer.

Because the PSA test is not completely reliable as far as its predictive value, a patient with a high PSA level may not necessarily have cancer; and a patient with a very low PSA may not be cancer free. In fact, high grade, more aggressive cancers can lose their resemblance to prostate cells altogether and may not even produce PSA. The PSA provides only a statistical approximation, and there are often exceptions. PSA results are discussed in terms of probabilities—the likelihood of prostate cancer being present, and the likelihood that it may have spread beyond the prostate gland.

I'm often suspicious of any PSA greater than 2.5, especially with men who are 40 to 55 years old; however, I'm equally suspicious of a patient who has a normal PSA or even a low PSA, but an abnormal digital rectal examination. For example, if you have a man who has a prostate nodule and his PSA is 1.2, that's worth looking into with further testing. It may become even more concerning if he tells you that his father had prostate cancer or his brother had prostate cancer at an early age, or if he's an African-American. These are all considerations.

Once the presence of cancer is confirmed, the PSA results can be used to estimate the approximate size of the tumor, and the extent of the dis-

What Factors Other Than Cancer Can Affect PSA Levels?

✓ Benign prostatic hyperplasia (BPH)

✓ Infection (prostatitis)

✓ Trauma such as biopsy or overly vigorous digital rectal examination (DRE)

✓ Ejaculation (up to a 40% elevation, returning to normal within 48 hours)

✓ Strenuous exercise involving the buttocks or perineum (such as bicycle riding)

✓ Medical procedures such as balloon dilation of the prostate, transrectal ultrasound-guided biopsy, and transurethral resection of the prostate (TURP)

✓ Medications such as finasteride (Proscar or Propecia) used to treat BPH can decrease PSA levels by as much as 50 percent.

✓ PC-SPECS and other herbal mixtures marketed "for prostate health" may also affect PSA levels.

ease. The higher the PSA the more likely it is that the tumor is large and the cancer has extended beyond the prostate. Again, there are exceptions. Some patients with a high PSA may have small, curable cancers. Some men with a low PSA may have more advanced disease. Even with the exceptions and inaccuracies, the PSA test remains the most valuable tool available for diagnosing and monitoring prostate cancer.

The most important factor in deciding on treatment is whether or not the cancer has *metastasized,* that is, spread to parts of the body beyond the prostate. The higher the PSA value, the larger a tumor is likely to be, and the greater the likelihood that the cancer has spread outside the prostate capsule. Taken together, the PSA and DRE tests are very useful for detecting cancer, but they provide only rough estimates of how far the disease has actually progressed. As discussed later in this chapter, more tests are necessary to determine the precise *stage* and *grade* of the disease. Staging and grading are standard systems for classifying the disease, that is, for evaluating the nature or grade of the malignancy, and the extent of the disease. All of this information is critical for deciding which treatment options are available for each patient.

Before having a biopsy, you should have your PSA tested several times at the same laboratory. There can be considerable variation with PSA test results depending on the lab and the particular test used. The FDA has approved a number of PSA tests, or assays, produced by various manu-facturers; however, most of these tests have been approved only for PSA monitoring, not for diagnosis. Test results can vary by as much as 8 to 10 percent even when the test is done by the same laboratory. This variation is not considered significant, but it is important for patients to try to have their annual PSA test performed by the same lab each year, or at least to use the same FDA-approved brand of test.

Patients are advised to check with their local laboratory to find out what brand of PSA test is being used. Be sure the particular test at your lab has been FDA-approved for *both* diagnosis and monitoring of prostate cancer (some tests are approved only for monitoring). At our institution, we have implemented an advanced in-house blood lab that employs the Immulite assay series produced by Diagnositic Products Corporation (DPC). These state of the art tests utilize a process known as *enzyme-amplified chemi-luminescence,* which allows for highly sensitive PSA readings. One of the advantages of Immulite is greater precision as far as the number of deci-mal places reported (ie. to a level of 0.005 ng/ml). While not yet widely available, the Immulite assays are currently the most accurate PSA tests with FDA approval for diagnosis and for monitoring.

Why is There Controversy About the PSA Test?

Critics of PSA screening contend that the test detects many incidental, non-aggressive cancers that don't need to be diagnosed or treated because such cancers will never become life-threatening for the patient. The crit-ics argue that many patients are being tested and treated unnecessarily. They also point out that no studies have proven that any of the curative treatments for prostate cancer improve survival. There are several ongoing studies to evaluate survival benefits of treatment, but they are still years from completion. Even though the overall impact of treatment on survival is not yet conclusively established, researchers have compiled extensive data (based on PSA monitoring and biopsy) to ascertain cure rates for each treatment modality.

Much of the controversy centers on the medical value of PSA screening and its cost-effectiveness. Critics are correct in pointing out that the PSA reports a significant percentage of "false positives," though at our institution we are finding less than about 10 percent of men with PSA readings over 10 do not have cancer. Some of these men will suffer the anxiety, inconvenience, and expense of further testing in order to rule out cancer. The fact remains that these tests can save many lives, and therefore, the cost and inconvenience appears to be justified. Although doctors have a difficult time distinguishing between cancers that are aggressive and those that are clinically insignificant, all prostate cancers are potentially life-threatening. Once prostate cancer is diagnosed, doctors have a responsibility to make their patients aware of their treatment options and the risks involved.

Critics argue that as many as 30 percent of men over the age of 50 have cancers that are insignificant, that will grow slowly and never cause any problem during their lifetimes. According to this argument, there is no point in diagnosing or treating these cancers. The fact is, however, that most prostate cancers diagnosed with PSA testing are clinically significant, and are potentially life-threatening. In a study conducted on men who were autopsied, no patient with a PSA greater than 4 had cancer that was clinically incidental. Moreover, in some men who appear to have incidental cancers, the disease will develop later, and they may eventually die of their cancer. The only way the large number of annual prostate cancer deaths is likely to be reduced is with early detection and treatment.

With that said, it should be emphasized that every man must make his own personal choice of whether to be tested for prostate cancer; and those patients who are diagnosed with the disease have the right to make the decision of whether or not to be treated. While there is no single treatment or set of answers for all patients, each man can make informed decisions about diagnosis and treatment.

What is PSA Velocity?

PSA velocity refers to the rate of change of the PSA over time. The measurement of PSA velocity is known as PSAV or PSA slope. The assumption is that the annual rate of change of the PSA value for men with cancer is greater than for men without cancer, both those with normal prostate glands and those with BPH. A rise in the PSA of 0.75 or more in a year may be an indicator of cancer. A rise in the PSA less than 0.75 might indicate BPH, or could be a fluctuation attributed to a normal prostate.

Studies have shown that the use of PSA velocity can reduce the number of unnecessary biopsies. For patients with BPH, the number of biopsies may be reduced from 40 percent to 10 percent. PSA velocity can be especially telling for patients whose PSA is within the normal range but increasing rapidly. For example, a patient whose PSA rises from 1.3 to 2.3 to 3.7 over a period of two years might have a cancer detectable with a biopsy even before his PSA climbs above the normal limit of 4.0. This is where the benefit of early detection becomes most obvious, as the cancer can be caught when it is most treatable.

PSA velocity is also useful in diagnosing those patients whose PSA values are in the grey area between 4 and 10, and who have negative biopsies. For example, a patient with a 5.8 PSA value and negative biopsy might undergo another biopsy the following year if his PSA climbs significantly. An increase in PSA of less than 0.75 may rule out the need for another biopsy. The measurement of the PSA values over time greatly increases the ability of a doctor to make an accurate clinical diagnosis. For best results, the patient is usually advised to have his PSA tested at least three times over a period of two years.

While the PSA test can be very important, and may be the single most important marker to determine the likelihood of cancer being present, the PSA alone may not be as important as the PSA velocity. The history of the patient's PSA over time also enables us obtain the doubling time (PSADT) —the amount of time it takes for the PSA value to double—which can help us determine how rapidly the cancer is growing. A PSADT of less than 12 years and a PSA velocity greater than 0.75 indicate greater likelihood of malignancy.

What Are Free and Bound PSA?

Several other approaches for measuring PSA levels can allow us to make a more accurate diagnosis. Among these are free (or unbound) versus bound (or complexed) PSA. These terms refer to the fact that PSA appears in the bloodstream in two distinct molecular forms, either unattached to other substances (free), or combined with other protein molecules (bound). The percent-free PSA test measures how much PSA circulates free in the bloodstream compared to the total PSA level. The percentage of free PSA tends to be lower in men who have prostate cancer than in men who do not.

Some studies indicate that the amount of bound PSA in the blood is higher when cancer is present, while the amount of free PSA is higher in men with BPH. The percent-free PSA test is especially useful for diagnosing patients whose PSA falls into the grey area between 4 and 10, and even at lower levels between 2.5 and 4—when it is most difficult to distinguish cancer from benign enlargement of the prostate (BPH). By increasing the accuracy of PSA testing in this way, the number of unnecessary biopsies can be reduced. The percent-free PSA test may also be a valuable asset for monitoring patients after treatment.

What is PSA Density?

Another way we can sometimes distinguish between cancer and BPH is by measuring the PSA density, which is the PSA value divided by the volume of the prostate gland, as determined by transrectal ultrasound (discussed below). For a man with an enlarged prostate, the PSA value should not be greater than 15% of the weight of the prostate. Anything higher than that may be indicative of prostate cancer. The measurement of PSA density can help determine which men with slightly elevated PSA values should be subjected to biopsies to confirm or rule out the presence of cancer.

What is the PAP test?

At our institution, a PAP (Prostatic Acid Phosphatase) blood test is also routinely performed, as this test has been demonstrated by myself as well as others in the medical literature to be perhaps the single most adverse feature associated with prostate cancer. Before the advent of the PSA test, the

PAP test was the only prostate tumor marker. In fact, doctors believed that the test was so accurate that if the patient had an elevated PAP, he should not undergo surgery because he would predictably have cancer beyond the prostate capsule, and therefore could not be cured by surgery.

After the advent of the PSA test and with the general excitement over the PSA marker, the PAP became less and less used. However, we never stopped using it and have even found that this test can be an independent prognosticator for treatment failure. In other words, in patients undergoing radiation therapy, we found that the PAP was as important as the PSA, and possibly more important for patients with advanced cancer, so we routinely employ it. Similar to radiation data, the PAP also carries tremendous statistical power for predicting whether or not a patient will relapse after surgery. Recent studies are finding that in patients with an elevated PAP, over 85% of those patients are going to fail after surgery. This should be no surprise in view of older pre-PSA surgical data.

What is a Prostate Biopsy?

A prostate biopsy is a procedure by which samples of tissue are removed from suspicious areas of the prostate gland for microscopic examination by a pathologist. A biopsy is absolutely necessary to confirm the presence of cancer and should be undertaken prior to any treatment of the disease. The biopsy also provides us with a wealth of information about the specific characteristics of the cancer.

When performing a biopsy, the doctor will use an imaging technique called transrectal ultrasound (TRUS) for guidance in order to insert a narrow needle through the wall of the rectum into the prostate gland. Doctors can perform the biopsy through the perineum, the area between the rectum and scrotum. The needle removes a tiny core of tissue (usually measuring about 1/2-inch by 1/16-inch) that is sent to the laboratory to see if cancer is present. Although the procedure may sound painful, a biopsy usually causes little discomfort because an instrument called a biopsy gun inserts and removes the needle in a fraction of a second. In addition, a local anesthetic can be used to numb the area. The procedure can be performed in the doctor's office and usually takes only about 15 minutes.

The prostate biopsy has traditionally involved obtaining at least six core samples of tissue. This procedure, known as the sextant biopsy, draws tissue from the base, mid-gland and apex for a total of six core samples. Recent studies have shown that increasing the number of samples can significantly increase the detection of malignancy. The number of biopsy samples taken now ranges from 6 to 13 or more. The 5-region biopsy approach obtains additional samples from the mid-gland tissue and the lateral zones or lobes on each side of the gland.

Your biopsy report should indicate how many tissue samples were taken from specific areas of the prostate, and how many specimens showed cancer. The report should also indicate what percentage of each core contained cancer and how many specimens showed solid cores. If each core is solid, then the tumor is likely to be large. If the cores are small and scattered, the needle probably passed through small tumors. More than 50% cancer in any one core and/or multiple positive cores would suggest a larger tumor. When more than half of a prostate lobe is involved, the outlook is less optimistic because larger tumors have a less favorable prognosis. Your doctor will use all of this information about the size and extent of your cancer, along with the results of the rest of the work-up tests, to develop a strategy for treating the disease.

Recent studies have shown that biopsies guided by the color-flow Doppler ultrasound imaging technique (see discussion below) have the advantage of showing the optimal sites from which to secure tissue samples. Once the initial diagnosis has been established, I typically request that the specimen slides be reviewed by a pathologist who specializes in prostate pathology. Specialists in evaluating prostate biopsy specimens are available at a number of labs and major medical centers. Samples can be sent to these specialists for "second opinions," as the pathological interpretation can vary. There is an "art" to interpreting the slides, and it is that interpretation that your doctor will use in determining how to best treat the disease.

What is the Gleason Score?

Under the microscope, prostate cancer cells exhibit a particular range of aggressiveness, from slow-growing to fast-growing, and they are ranked accordingly. The ranking used to identify how aggressive or abnormal a cancer appears is called the Gleason scale. The scale essentially runs from

2 to 10, with the least aggressive tumors at the low end and the fastest growing, more aggressive tumors at the high end of the scale.

Slow-growing tumors appear similar to normal tissue and are called "well-differentiated." Fast-growing cancers appear abnormal and are called "poorly differentiated." Between the two extremes are cancers which are classified as moderately differentiated." The Gleason system defines five glandular patterns of cancerous cell tissue, from completely differentiated to completely undifferentiated. Tumors often possess more than one cellular pattern, and therefore, both primary and secondary patterns are graded. The two grades are combined to get the actual Gleason score, ranging from 2 (1 + 1) to 10 (5 + 5), with most cancers falling somewhere in between (See Figure 5).

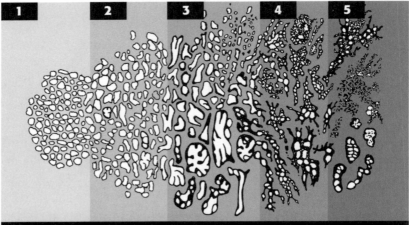

Figure 5—A simplified drawing of the Gleason grading system, showing the five distinct grades of cancerous tissue, as seen under low magnification. The two most common cell patterns seen in the tissue sample are added together to arrive at a Gleason score.

The higher the Gleason score, the more likely it is that the cancer is more aggressive and has already spread beyond the prostate capsule or metastasized to other parts of the body. Unfortunately, like the PSA scale, the Gleason scale provides only an approximation of how aggressive a cancer is and how likely it is that the cancer has spread. One part of the prostate gland may appear to be more aggressive or abnormal than other parts, and there is some element of chance as to where exactly the needle obtains each specimen.

The imprecision of Gleason scoring creates exceptions when interpreting the numbers. Some men with high Gleason scores may have small, curable cancers, while other men with lower numbers may have cancers that are more advanced. Nevertheless, the Gleason score is fairly accurate in predicting how aggressive the cancer is and how rapidly it will spread.

What is Transrectal Ultrasound (TRUS)?

Technically referred to a *transrectal ultrasonography*, this is a technique that projects sound waves off the prostate and surrounding organs to create an image. The sound waves are generated by a probe placed inside the rectum. Transrectal ultrasound imaging can in many cases accurately identify the local spread of cancer through the prostate capsule. In some cases, however, areas of cancer growth through the prostatic capsule may be too small to be visible. As mentioned, ultrasound is often used to guide the biopsy needle to suspicious sites in the prostate. The technique is also used for real time guidance in conjunction with seed implants, external radiation therapy, and other treatments.

At our institution, color-flow Doppler ultrasound is utilized since it provides enhanced visualization and greater definition compared to the conventional gray-scale technique. While there is an art to interpreting color-flow Doppler images, tumors tend to demonstrate increased blood perfusion or *hypervascularity* as findings consistent with malignancy. Tumors are growing faster than normal prostate cells and require more blood to nurture their growth. Tumors therefore tend to create blood vessels around them as they grow, and these can be identified by color-flow Doppler ultrasound. A conventional TRUS typically shows what are called *hypoechogenic* areas, which are darker shades of gray. A color-flow Doppler ultrasound may show the same image, but it provides additional insight into how much perfusion of blood is going into the region, and can reveal whether just one prostate nodule is involved or if there is more cancer dispersed throughout the gland (See Color Inset, Figures 1-B, 1-C, 1-D).

What is a CT Scan?

The CT scan (also called CAT scan) uses *computer tomography* to produce a 3-dimensional image of the prostate and surrounding organs. CT scans rely on computer-reconstructed x-rays to give a cross-sectional view of the body. A CT scan through the pelvis reveals the outline of the prostate.

CT scans can identify prostate enlargement and show the size and shape of the gland, but it is not as effective for assessing the extent of cancer or visualizing cancer within the gland itself. While CT scans provide less defined images of the outer prostatic contour and internal architecture, CT images do accurately delineate the spatial relationship between the prostate, rectum and pubic bones. More contemporary spiral or helical CT scans provide greater resolution while taking less time to acquire the information.

What is an Endorectal MRI?

MRI refers to *magnetic resonance imaging,* a state of the art technique that generates a magnetic field, which harmlessly reacts with the tissues of the body to produce a distinct and complex image of internal organs. The endorectal MRI utilizes a rectal probe to provide sharper images and is especially useful in detecting capsular penetration. The MRI is primarily used in staging biopsy-proven prostate cancer. This imaging technique is more accurate than CT scans or standard grey-scale ultrasound for detecting cancer that has penetrated the prostate capsule. However, approximately 30% of patients who do not show capsular penetration with MRI may still have some penetration that is too small to be detected.

While its availability is limited to only a few institutions in the U.S., magnetic resonance spectroscopic imaging (MRSI) is the most discriminating test in terms of both the internal architecture of the prostate gland and determining whether or not the cancer has spread beyond the prostate capsule, which is termed *extracapsular extension* (EPE). With its high degree of detail, the endorectal MRI can show whether or not there is rectal or seminal vesicle involvement. Bladder invasion can also be detected by an endorectal MRI, while it's not commonly seen with a CT scan or with a conventional grey-scale ultrasound study.

The endorectal MRI is much like an ultrasound probe in that it is placed in the rectum and allows you to image the prostate very closely. It's as detailed a test as you can get in terms of looking at the capsule of the prostate and determining whether or not there is cancer that has extended outside of the prostate capsule. Approximately 90% of our patients undergo an endorectal MRI (preferably MRSI) prior to treatment. The only reason a patient wouldn't have an MRI is if his insurance company would not pay for it and the patient can't afford the test, as it is expensive. The cost of a diagnostic pelvic MRI is at least two to three times higher than the cost for a TRUS or CT scan.

What is a Bone Scan?

A bone scan is an imaging technique used to detect bone metastases, which appear as "hot spots" on film. It is far more sensitive than conventional x-rays. The bone scan procedure is performed by injecting a small amount of radioactive dye called *technetium* into the patient's bloodstream. A special camera is then used to photograph the skeleton, and any irritation of the bone will show up as a spot on the image.

If a patient's PSA is high, greater than 10, or if the Gleason score is greater than or equal to 7, then I usually recommend a bone scan. A spot on a bone scan may be caused by cancer that has metastasized, or by arthritis and other causes. When an abnormality shows up on a bone scan, further tests such as traditional x-rays or a CT scan may be used to determine if the cause is cancer. It is important to establish a "base-line" to differentiate between cancer and other abnormalities.

What is a ProstaScint™ Scan?

ProstaScint™ is a staging test that utilizes a radioactive isotope, which is attached to a *monoclonal antibody* (mAb), which targets a specific cancer protein know as *prostate specific membrane antigen* (PSMA). After this combined isotope-mAb is injected into the bloodstream, it will track down that particular cancer protein and then attaches to it. This is an imaging test rather than a blood test per se. Three to four days after being injected, a patient is scanned with a special camera that picks up the radiation emitted by the isotope and locates the cancer.

If a patient's PSA is very high, for example, in excess of 20, or if there are other additional factors like a Gleason score of 8 or higher, or an elevated PAP, then a patient should probably undergo a Prostascint™ study. I use this test for patients whom I suspect are at a high risk for having cancer which has gone beyond the prostate gland. The Prostascint™ studies may lend some important information for these patients because it tells us a great deal about soft tissue. If there is lymph node involvement, a Prostascint™ scan may show the cancer going very accurately and methodically from the prostate gland up to the internal iliac or lymph node chain, or to known sites or banks where prostate cancer commonly goes.

As yet, not many institutions use the Prostascint™ scan although its availability is growing and it is FDA approved. It can be a revealing test, but again, it should be limited to patients having more aggressive cancer. I wouldn't put everyone through it since it's associated with false positives and it's expensive. One of its advantages, however, is that while other tests may be affected by a patient being on hormones, the Prostascint™ scan should still be predictably effective because it's looking for PSMA rather than PSA. Compared to PSA, only relatively small amounts of PSMA are detectable in the bloodstream of prostate cancer patients.

Fusing the Prostascint™ with a helical CT study or MRI significantly improves the predictive accuracy of the Prostascint™ test (fewer false positives and negatives). In patients with Gleason 8 to 10 tumors, a Prostascint™ / CT / PET Fusion may be dictated. Fusion studies are relatively new and are only as good as the technologist performing it and the radiologist interpreting it. Like everything else in this field, it pays to search out experienced practitioners.

What is a Lymphadenectomy?

Lymphadenectomy or removal of lymph nodes, is a surgical procedure which looks at the lymph node-bearing sites that prostate cancer can drain to. As with any part of the body when cancer is present, there is always a station of lymph nodes where cancer can collect or accumulate. The lymph nodes are scavengers of abnormal things in the body. The prostate gland has its own stations of lymph nodes, the primary ones being the obturator lymph nodes and the internal iliac lymph nodes. These reside in the pelvis. Once the lymph nodes collect cancer, they often disperse the cancer into the blood stream.

My personal opinion is that an exploratory lymphadenectomy is a far more rigorous and invasive procedure than a relatively non-invasive primary treatment such as a seed implant. Urologists rarely do lymphadenec-tomies, because it is a morbid procedure in and of itself. I generally favor giving the patient the benefit of the doubt by doing an implant, barring obvious metastases to the lymph nodes or obvious lymph node spread, as determined by radiographic studies. Given the fact that we are dem-onstrating successful treatment results even in patients who have lymph node spread, by using other combined treatment methods such as hor-monal therapies followed by sophisticated radiation techniques, lympha-dendectomies would add little but morbidity to the picture.

Laparoscopic lymph node dissection is a less invasive procedure than lymphadenectomy and may be more attractive, but the laparascopic pro-cedure is also less accurate. Nonetheless, if a Prostascint™ Fusion study is highly suggestive of lymph node involvement, directed laparascopic lymph node sampling may be useful.

What is Ploidy Analysis?

Another test sometimes performed by the pathologist utilizes a hi-tech examination called *flow cytometry* to analyze the nuclear DNA content, or *DNA Ploidy,* of cancer cells. Samples for analysis may be obtained from bi-opsy or operating tissue. The genetic information derived from this test al-lows cancer cells to be classified as "diploid," "tetraploid," or "aneuploid."

Aneuploid cancers generally have a less favorable prognosis than dip-loid cancers, and if left untreated are more likely to progress rapidly. Dip-loid cancers have a more favorable prognosis than either aneuploid or tetraploid. Why ploidies differ and why some indicate a more aggressive cancer than others remains the subject of continuing research.

While this method of analysis is very sensitive, the predictive value of flow cytometry is not definitive, and the test is not reliable enough to be used by itself as a diagnostic tool. As far as determining the aggressiveness of the tumor, ploidy can be enhanced when combined with the patient's PSA and Gleason score. It is a subject of debate whether the data on ploidy is solid enough to be used as a basis for treatment decisions. Most physicians do not rely on this form of testing and consider it investiga-tional. When ploidy is used, it is most often called for when the patient's Gleason score is greater than or equal to 7. Some studies have suggested that if the PSA is greater than or equal to 15, and if the ploidy is aneuploid, then the likelihood is that the cancer will already have metastasized.

What Other Tests are Commonly Used?

Depending on the specifics of the case, a number of other tests may be utilized and are commonly used in my practice. Their names may sound like alphabet soup, but they are all useful in determining the extent and aggressiveness of the cancer. Don't be put off by the medical terminology. Patients should not be reluctant to discuss with their doctors the purpose of each of these laboratory tests as they relate to their own individual cases.

Some of these tests, or *markers,* may be used to identify mutant tumor populations, or aggressive tumors in patients without elevated PSAs. Markers of this type include NSE (Neuron Specific Enolase), CGA (Chromagranin A), and CEA (Carcinoembryonic Antigen). A number of other lab tests help to determine whether or not some form of hormonal therapy may be indicated either in the short term or at a later date. These tests include those that measure levels of Testosterone (total and bio-available), DHT (dihydrotestosterone), DHEA-S (dehyrdoepiandrosterone sulphate), Estradiol, Prolactin, LH (Luteinizing Hormone) and Androstenedione.

Other evaluative procedures, such as Urine Pyrilinks-D™ (Dpd), N-telopeptide (serum or urine), and Bone Specific Alkaline Phosphatase, are often used in addition to a Bone Mineral Density (BMD) test to establish a baseline for bone integrity. This is especially important for patients undergoing hormonal therapy, which can cause bone loss or resorption. With regard to the BMD test, in my practice, a quantitative computerized tomography (QCT) scan is preferred over the Dual Energy X-ray Absorptiometry (DEXA) scan, as the QCT provides more accurate results. Additional tests such as a urine cytology study and NMP-22 bladder cancer marker may be used to evaluate for other malignancies. Tests such as IGF-1 and IL-6 may be included in a systemic evaluation.

There are other areas within the pathology itself which we may want to examine. Whether or not a cancer has attached itself to a nerve *(perineural invasion or PNI)* is important because we know that a nerve typically tracks throughout the gland and outside of the gland, and that it can act as something of a conduit for the cancer. Perineural invasion essentially allows the cancer to get a free ride outside the prostate gland proper. When pathological examination indicates extensive PNI, there is an increased likelihood of extra-prostatic extension, such as capsular penetration and/or seminal vesicle involvement. In addition, genetic markers like bcl2, p27, p53, and MIB-1 may help to determine the aggressiveness of tumors. These markers are obtained from immuno-histochemical stains from the initial tumor block (biopsied tissue).

CHAPTER THREE

CONSIDERATIONS PRIOR TO TREATMENT

How Much Time is There to Make a Decision About Treatment?

If you are a newly diagnosed patient, you should not be concerned that the several weeks which may be required for testing and consultations with your doctor will give the cancer time to grow and spread. In most cases, prostate cancer is slow to progress, as indicated by the slow rise of PSA values over time. In fact, by the time most men are diagnosed, they have already had the disease for several years. Judging by the slow rise of PSA levels, a newly diagnosed patient should be able to safely devote a month or so to becoming informed about the disease and learning about his treatment options. It is extremely unlikely that investing that amount of time will decrease the likelihood of a man being cured.

There may be rare exceptions to such a time frame when a patient's PSA doubling time is only 3 to 6 months, with a PSA of greater than 20 and a Gleason score of 8 to 10. With such a rapidly growing, aggressive cancer, the situation may warrant more expeditious research to determine the best treatment option, which should be undertaken without lengthy delays.

What is the Difference Between Early Stage and Metastatic Disease?

Deciding which treatments are appropriate in large part depends on the stage or extent of the cancer as indicated by the results of the work-up tests. The evaluation of stage is based on the doctor's interpretation of the test results. Different types of treatment are available as options for each patient depending on whether the cancer is locally confined to the prostate gland and nearby tissues, or whether the cancer has metastasized to distant parts of the body.

Early stage prostate cancer refers to small and medium size tumors that are most likely to be totally confined within the prostate. This stage is sometimes called *organ-confined disease* (OCD). *Locally advanced disease* is defined as cancer that has spread beyond the confines of the prostate proper (e.g. a bulky tumor extending into the periprostatic tissue or invading the seminal vesicles, bladder or rectum. The term *metastatic disease* indicates that the cancer has spread to the regional lymph nodes or distant sites such as bone, lungs or liver.

In the case of metastatic disease, microscopic clumps of cancer cells break away from the original tumor and travel via the bloodstream or lymph system to another location of the body, where new tumors start to grow. These metastatic tumors, wherever they have formed, are made of the same kind of cells as the original tumor. Prostate cancer that has spread to the bones does not become bone cancer. It is prostate cancer outside the prostate, and needs to be treated accordingly.

As the cancerous growth expands, it presses on surrounding tissues and replaces healthy cells at the perimeter of the mass. As it grows in size, symptoms of the disease will eventually start to appear. These vary depending on the site and nature of the cancer. Metastatic disease will typically extend to the regional lymph nodes, and then to the bones of the hip or lower back. While the likelihood of cure is very small, advanced disease can be treated in order to slow the progression of the cancer and to relieve symptoms. We have had considerable success treating patients with minimal to modest pelvic lymph node involvement when compared to those having extensive lymph node metastases.

What are the Stages of Prostate Cancer?

A staging system is a standardized way to classify the extent to which the disease has spread. Decades of studies have led to the classification of prostate cancer into essentially four distinct stages. These were initially identified as A, B, C, and D in the Whitmore-Jewett system, which dates from 1956. There are sub-stages for each stage of prostate cancer as well.

The stage is based on factors such as the size or volume of disease, Gleason grade, and spread of disease beyond the prostate or to other sites in the body, such as the seminal vesicles, pelvic lymph nodes, or more distant sites such as lungs or bones. Accurate staging of the disease is crucial to developing an appropriate treatment plan.

Since 1992, most physicians have switched over to a newer staging system known as TNM (tumor, nodes, metastases) that describes the extent of the primary tumor (in stages ranging from Tl through T4), whether the cancer has invaded the regional lymph nodes (N stage), and whether the cancer has metastasized (M stage). The TNM system roughly parallels the A to D classification system, but the TNM system subdivides each stage in more detail. The TNM system has been revised over the years, and the most recent is that which appears in the 2002 staging manual of the American Joint Committee on Cancer (AJCC).

The stages are classified as follows:

T Stages: There are two types of T classifications. The *clinical stage* is an assessment made on the basis of clinical tests performed without direct examination of the tumor or cancer cells. The classifications described in this section are primarily based on clinical evaluation. Although the tests used in staging are always undergoing improvement, clinical staging is a subjective process, and therefore, not foolproof. Staging tests provide valuable information to the physician, but unavoidable errors in assessing the stage still do occur. The *pathological stage* provides more precise and verifiable data on the extent of the disease. It is accomplished by means of biopsy and surgical exploration.

Stage T1 (also known as Stage A): These are cancers confined to the prostate that cannot be felt during rectal examination and produce no symptoms. These tumors usually cannot be seen with ultrasound or other imaging techniques. Stage T1 tumors are often found by accident during routine examination of tissue removed during surgery for benign prostatic hypertrophy (BPH). As many as 10% of men who undergo transurethral resection of the prostate

(TURP) for BPH are discovered to have unsuspected prostate cancer. This stage is further divided into three sub-stages.

Stage T1a: Although there is some variance in definitions of this sub-stage, it typically describes a "focalized tumor" (spherical and possessing a distinct boundary between the tumor and surrounding tissue) that comprises 5% or less of the surgical specimen.

Stage T1b: Typically a "diffuse tumor" that comprises over 5% of the removed specimen of prostate tissue. Note that T1a and T1b are stages which are most often detected incidentally following a TURP.

Stage T1c: The tumor is not palpable and usually identified by biopsy performed after determination of an elevated PSA.

Stage T2 (also know as Stage B): The tumor can be felt by rectal examination, but is still confined to the prostate gland.

Stage T2a: The tumor is palpable and involves less than one half of one side or lobe of the prostate.

Stage T2b: The cancer is palpable and involves more than one half of one lobe but not both lobes of the prostate gland.

Stage T2c: The cancer is palpable and involves both lobes.

Stage T3 and T4 (also known as Stage C): These are tumors that have extended through the prostatic capsule (extracapsular extension), and are no longer confined to the prostate. Stage T3 and T4 cancers often involve most or all of the prostate gland, and the entire prostate may feel hard upon rectal examination.

Stage T3a: The tumor has extended through the prostatic capsule on one side or two sides (unilateral or bilateral extracapsular extension).

Stage T3b: The cancer has spread to the seminal vesicles. Often symptoms of the disease will begin to appear at this stage, such as difficulty urinating.

Stage T4: The tumor has invaded structures adjacent to the prostate other than the seminal vesicles.

Stage T4a: The tumor has invaded the bladder neck, rectum or external sphincter.

Stage T4b: The tumor has invaded the levator muscles and/or is fixed to the pelvic wall.

N Stages: These stages describe regional lymph node involvement.

Stage NX: Indicates the regional lymph nodes have not been assessed.

Stage N0: Indicates the cancer has not spread to the lymph nodes.

Stage N1 (also known as Stage D1): The cancer has spread beyond the prostate and invaded the regional lymph nodes.

M Stages: These stages describe distant metastasis.

MX: Indicates distant metastasis cannot be assessed.

M0: Indicates there is no distant metastasis.

M1 (also known as Stage D2): The cancer has spread to distant sites in the body. Metastatic disease will often spread to nearby bones, but may also involve the liver, lungs or other tissues.

M1a: Indicates non-regional lymph node involvement.

M1b: Indicates cancer that has spread to the bones.

M1c: Indicates cancer that has spread to other sites with or without bone disease.

As indicated by biopsy and surgical exploration, pathological stages include the following:

pT2: Organ confined

pT2a: Unilateral

pT2b: Bilateral

pT3: Extraprostatic extension

pT3a: Extraprostatic extension

pT3b: Seminal vesicle invasion

pT4: Invasion of bladder, rectum

As discussed in the previous chapter, there are a wide variety of staging tests, each possessing unique capabilities and serving a specific function in the staging process. Some tests are used to visualize the internal structures of the body, such as the CT scan, ultrasound (especially 3-D color-flow Doppler TRUS), endorectal MRI (magnetic resonance imaging,) or 3D-MRSI (three dimensional, magnetic resonance spectrographic imaging). These techniques allow doctors to improve their assessment of cancer location and extent within the prostate.

Other tests are used to identify the presence of cancer in various parts of the body, such as the chest x-ray or bone scan. Blood tests such as the PSA and PAP may be used to give a general indication of the extent and aggressiveness of the disease. These tests can be used for preliminary staging and for subsequent staging to track changes in a patient's illness or evaluate the effectiveness of treatment.

What Factors Determine Low, Intermediate and High Risk Patients?

Low-risk patients would be characterized as those having clinical T1 (non-palpable disease), low volume malignancy found in the biopsy specimens (e.g. less than 50% core involvement), a Gleason score of less than or equal to 6, serum PSA less than or equal to 10 and a non-elevated PAP. In addition, the endorectal MRI or spectroscopic MRI and color-flow Doppler ultrasound should not demonstrate more extensive tumor than was anticipated.

In view of the fact that at our institution we treat both intermediate and high risk patients similarly, these patients are routinely grouped together. They may have a clinical stage tumor which is greater than or equal to T2B, a PSA greater than 10, Gleason score greater than or equal to 7 and/or an elevated PAP. Intermediate risk patients typically have only one of these risk factors, while high risk patients possess two or more. If a PSA is extremely high or if a PAP is very high, I have found that generally means that the cancer has left the prostate gland, although it may not mean that it has spread widely into the bloodstream, but may be suggestive of cancer spreading to tissues around the prostate and/or the lymph nodes (locally advanced disease). These patients are still curable.

Other tests and factors are also taken into account when assessing risk. Evidence of perineural invasion and/or ploidy status (for example, an aneuploid tumor) may predict a less favorable prognosis, and as such, patients having these features are most commonly treated in the intermediate to high-risk category. The same applies to other adverse indicators such as the suppressor gene p27 and the monoclonal antibody MIB1. Genes that relate to tumor growth (oncogenes) such as bcl-2 and growth factors obtained in serum analysis such as TGF beta-1 may also portend more aggressive, higher risk cancers. While these clinical, laboratory, pathology and radiology findings may sound like complicated medical jargon, they are actually crucial pieces of information that your doctor can use to create a profile of the cancer that will help you in making the difficult decisions about treatment.

As indicated previously, a patient's treatment options in large part depend on exactly how far the cancer has spread. Accurate staging allows us to determine the probability of whether or not the cancer has escaped the prostate capsule. There are a number of powerful tools that enable us to predict which patients—those having certain clinical stages, PSA levels and Gleason scores—may harbor extracapsular extension (cancer that has escaped the prostate capsule) as well as lymph node involvement. These tools are statistical approaches to risk assessment that allow doctors and patients to know what to expect given their individual test results. The statistical calculations are based on data found in peer-reviewed medical literature that relate various disease indices (such as stage, PSA and Gleason scores) to outcomes reported with each type of treatment.

One of these risk assessment tools is called the Partin Tables, named after its originator, Dr. Alan Partin, of Johns Hopkins University. The Partin Tables are based on problem-solving "algorithm" procedures, a series of complex analyses and formulas for assessing a patient's risk. Using this statistical approach, patients are able to plug their own data into formulas that reveal the probability of the cancer being confined to the prostate. The tables also predict the likelihood of extracapsular penetration, as well as lymph node and seminal vesicle involvement. Researchers developed the Partin Tables by analyzing thousands of pathology specimens taken at the time of surgery and comparing those results with the initial PSA levels, Gleason scores and stages.

The Partin Tables don't take into account every risk factor and cannot predict cure, but they do provide an estimate of the extent of the cancer that can help doctors and patients determine which treatment options are appropriate based on the specifics of each individual case. Patients with the highest probability that the cancer has not yet spread beyond the prostate are considered the best candidates for surgery as well as other curative treatment options such as radiation therapy. Calculations based on the Partin Tables for any individual patient are not 100% accurate, but they do provide us with a valuable assessment of the probability as to how far the cancer may have spread based on a large numbers of patients.

The Partin Tables are available through the Prostate Cancer Research Institute's web site located at www.pcri.org, and are part of a computer software application called Prostate Cancer Tools II. This web site provides a number of related tools that can help a patient analyze the likely outcomes of his specific case with regard to not only the surgical option but also with regard to external beam radiation therapy, brachytherapy, and various combination therapies that are discussed in the chapters ahead.

CHAPTER FOUR

TREATMENT OPTIONS

What are the Most Common Treatments for Prostate Cancer?

The various treatment alternatives for prostate cancer are at present classified as "curative" or "palliative." Those patients who have early stage prostate cancer are candidates for curative treatments. In the past, the treatment options for such patients had been limited to surgery (radical prostatectomy) and radiation therapy, like that used with many other forms of cancer. Both treatment modalities have seen significant advances in recent years. In addition, a number of other techniques have been developed for the treatment of early stage prostate cancer. These include cryosurgery and therapies using protons and neutrons. While some therapies remain investigational, these more recent developments have given men a wider range of alternatives than ever before.

Those patients with late stage disease, or disease that has spread beyond the prostate gland, are generally considered incurable using presently available techniques. Some of you reading this book may fall into this category. But if you have late stage prostate cancer, there is no reason to give up hope simply because the medical community presently considers your condition incurable. Prostate cancer is often a very unpredictable disease, and the fact is that many men even with metastatic disease have lived for a decade or more with little or no progression of the cancer. Many eventually die of natural causes. And there are even the rare instances of spontaneous remission.

More importantly for patients with late stage prostate cancer, there are several treatment options including hormonal therapies that can be successfully used to slow or halt progression of the disease and to alleviate symptoms. Experimentation into the efficacy of a wide array of drugs and anti-cancer agents is also underway, any one of which may turn out to be the key to an improved form of treatment. And as research continues, one day in the not too distant future we may very well find a cure for any and all stages of prostate cancer.

A comprehensive list of treatment options and guidelines for cancer care professionals has been published by the National Comprehensive Cancer Network (NCCN), which includes specialists from 19 leading medical centers in the U.S. The guidelines are available from the American Cancer Society's National Cancer Information Center (1-800-ACS-2345), from the ACS web site (www.cancer.org) and the NCCN telephone information center (1-888-909-NCCN).

What Should a Patient Consider When Choosing a Treatment?

To get a handle on the basics of your case, you will need to find out from your doctor the following: 1) how much cancer you have, 2) where the cancer is located, and 3) how aggressive the cancer is. After your cancer has been graded and staged, you still have a lot to consider before deciding on treatment. As you begin to weigh your options with your doctor, you will want to take into account the following:

- ✔ Your age and life expectancy.
- ✔ Your overall health and any other serious medical conditions you may have.
- ✔ The stage, grade and risk factors associated with your cancer.
- ✔ The likelihood of cure with each type of treatment.
- ✔ Your concerns about the possible side effects associated with treatment.

Deciding on the best treatment and choosing the right doctor can be difficult. There are a number of legitimate treatment options, and each has its pros and cons. A persuasive argument can often be made for more than one option for which you may be eligible. To choose between treatments, you should carefully consider the likelihood of cure and the potential complications of each form of therapy. These are objective factors, but there are also equally important subjective factors relating to your personality, your priorities, emotional needs, and lifestyle.

Again, it is important to emphasize that each patient is different. Some men are extremely uncomfortable with the idea of having to live with side effects after treatment. Others are more concerned with survival issues than they are with quality of life considerations. You will want to find a balance that meets your personal needs and expectations. Ideally, your doctor will tailor a treatment plan that will minimize the impact of the disease while sparing you as much as possible from undesirable side effects of therapy.

In order to have confidence in your doctor's experience and expertise, you will need to find out how many patients he has treated and what his results have been with patients who are your age and have your PSA level and Gleason score. Your doctor should also be willing to provide you with a list of patients you can contact whose cases are similar to yours and who have undergone the type of treatment you are considering. Even with today's increased emphasis on privacy issues with regard to healthcare, many patients are willing to share their experiences with fellow patients. A doctor is more likely to refer you to men that he has treated successfully rather than to failures. But if you attend a support group meeting, you can ask those patients about their experiences with a particular treatment and/ or a particular doctor. Support group contact information and additional questions for your doctor are provided in the appendices of this book.

As you chart your course, keep accurate records of your lab tests and the results of all medical and therapeutic procedures. Making lists of your priorities and concerns about treatment can also be very useful. In the end, after learning all you can about your individual case and the pros and cons of each treatment, you should be able to make an educated decision about which treatment will be right for you. Keep in mind that each type of treatment is irreversible – once you have been treated, you can't undo it, so it's worth making every effort to think it through clearly from the beginning. In this situation, you are the one who ultimately has to be comfortable with the choice you make.

How are Treatments Compared?

As mentioned earlier, there are no modern randomized trials that compare the mainstream treatments like surgery, brachytherapy (radioactive implants) and external radiation. Instead, we rely on uncontrolled retrospective comparisons using PSA and Gleason categories to stratify patient groups according to low, intermediate and high risk; and then we compare the effectiveness of the various modalities. This represents a fairly reasonable form of analysis, given the overall prognostic consistency between institutions since the advent of PSA.

It should be emphasized that we are evaluating reported data and not mere opinions. It's true that the data requires interpretation, and statistics can be distorted to support a particular argument or specialty. But as more data is reported involving larger numbers of patients and longer follow-up (10 and 12 year studies), the areas where distortion and disagreement come into play are increasingly limited. As time goes on, the data becomes more and more persuasive. For example, there is a growing consensus among doctors that external radiation, brachytherapy and radical prostatectomy have about the same cure rates for the earliest stage prostate cancers, as demonstrated with those patients classified as low risk. While the cure rates may be comparable with this group of patients, the likelihood of side effects vary with each type of treatment, and therefore, quality of life also becomes an important consideration.

In comparing treatments, there is at least a grain of truth to the idea that we are dealing with an apples/oranges dilemma. Because each treatment modality has its own specific rationale and methodology, the reported results need to be scrutinized carefully, as each therapeutic specialty has its own criteria for measuring success and failure (see below "What is the definition of cure?"). Historically, there has been a bias in the medical literature and news media favoring surgery, but as we will see in the pages ahead, the most recent trends supported by the data have shifted the balance in favor of radiation, especially for intermediate and high risk patients.

You should also be aware that although statistics provide a general picture of what to expect from treatment, they may not be representative of present success rates. Over the past decade, improvements in all fields have increased the effectiveness of treatment. In some cases, the reported results may be out of date and not reflect the most recent innovations. For example, external radiation therapy has advanced in terms of accuracy and effectiveness as the technology has progressed from traditional external beam radiation therapy (EBRT) to 3-dimensional conformal radiation therapy (3-D CRT), both of which have been surpassed in just the past few years by Intensity Modulated Radiation Therapy (IMRT). Yet all three forms of radiation are still being utilized, and you will want to be sure exactly which type is offered by your doctor.

Finally, statistics are based on probabilities involving large numbers of patients. But as an individual, you are unique. And your case is just as unique. This is especially true when dealing with a disease as unpredictable as prostate cancer. There is always a possibility that what is true of most men may not be true for you.

What is the Definition of Cure?

Being cured of prostate cancer basically means the patient's entire cancer has been permanently eradicated. In practice, the methods that we use to determine which patients are cured have changed over the years. Before the advent of PSA monitoring, the only way for doctors to know whether any cancer was still present after treatment was if cancer was detected with a digital rectal examination or by repeated biopsies, or if metastases were found on a bone scan. With these limited means for determining the presence of cancer, many patients were mistakenly considered to be cured, when in fact they had residual cancers that were too small to be detected.

Patients whose cancers shrink after treatment to the point that they are undetectable are often described as being "in remission." But being in remission is not the same as being cured, because there is still some chance that these patients will have a recurrence of their cancer at some point in the future. Because prostate cancer progresses slowly, many patients in remission will die of other causes before their prostate cancer has time to re-grow. Before PSA testing, we couldn't be sure that a patient was really cured until about 10 to 15 years after treatment.

Since the introduction of PSA monitoring, we have been able to detect residual cancers much sooner after treatment. PSA results also showed us that cure rates were actually lower than previously believed for surgery and radiation, because of the number of residual cancers that had not been detected. This unexpected finding brought about a reappraisal of the entire field of prostate cancer therapy in the 1990's, at the same time spurring renewed progress by researchers working to improve the effectiveness of each type of treatment.

Soon after surgery, radiation therapy or cryosurgery, a patient's PSA will usually become undetectable or fall to very low levels. Most patients appear to be in remission shortly after being treated by any one of these curative therapies. The success of any treatment depends on achieving and maintaining a very low PSA endpoint. Some patients, however, will eventually show a rising PSA level if there is residual cancer. Such a PSA relapse is known as *biochemical failure*. Most patients who have residual cancer will show a rising PSA within five years of treatment. Most men whose PSA does not rise after five years are considered cured, but some additional men may experience a rising PSA even many years after treatment.

The ultimate cure rates for each treatment modality may take many years to determine. Cure rates are often illustrated by graphs showing the percentage of men without a rising PSA over time. The cure rate is established when we see the line of the graph flatten or "plateau" after a certain number of years, indicating a percentage of men who are most likely cured by a particular type of therapy (Figure 6). The medical term for this rigorous definition of cure is *biochemical disease-free survival* (bNED).

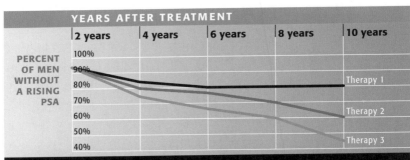

Figure 6—A graph showing the likelihood of biochemical disease survival for three hypothetical prostate cancer treatments as indicated by PSA. In this example, patients who underwent Therapy 1 showed a leveling off or plateau after about 5 years of treatment, indicating a cure rate of approximately 80%. Patients who were treated with Therapies 2 and 3 failed to plateau and continued to show additional men failing even 10 years after treatment, with the cure rate of Therapy 3 falling under 50%.

In actual practice, doctors often define cure using different PSA values for the endpoint or *nadir* level that should be reached after successful treatment. This discrepancy needs to be taken into account when interpreting the results for each type of therapy as reported by teams of researchers at different institutions. The specific PSA nadir values and definition of cure with each treatment modality will be noted in the pages ahead as we discuss each treatment option in more detail.

How does Treatment Affect Quality of Life?

In addition to cure rates, the efficacy of treatment is also evaluated in terms of the risk of complications, also referred to as *morbidity* or *toxicity*. All treatments for prostate cancer carry some risk of side effects that can have an impact on a patient's lifestyle or quality of life (QOL). Side effects may be temporary or permanent. By following up with patients after treatment through interviews and/or questionnaires, researchers attempt to measure the effects of therapy on lifestyle.

A common complication after treatment is erectile dysfunction, often referred to as impotence. Defined in practical terms as the inability to maintain an erection sufficient for intercourse, erectile dysfunction is a potential side effect from any therapy used to treat the prostate. The problem may be caused by damage to the nerves, blood vessels or tissues that normally allow the penis to fill with blood to form an erection.

Any large study of patients with long-term follow-up should take into account normal, age-related impotence, as there is a 1.5 % spontaneous decrease in potency with each year after the age of 40 (at age 40 only 80% have complete erectile function), and this is without any type of prostate treatment. Evaluating the effect of treatment on erectile function is made more problematical by the fact that prostate cancer typically affects an older age group for which there is a high incidence of sexual dysfunction prior to treatment. As many as 50% of prostate cancer patients already suffer from erectile dysfunction at the time they are diagnosed.

Another potential side effect of treatment is urinary incontinence, which may be caused by damage to the urethra, the bladder, and/or muscles that control urination. Urinary incontinence is often temporary, though some men experience permanent problems. Both the risk of urinary complications and the particular symptoms vary considerably depending on the type of treatment. Fortunately, there are a number of remedies available for correcting both erectile dysfunction and incontinence, thus enabling many men to maintain their quality of life after treatment.

CHAPTER FIVE

RADICAL SURGERY

What is a Radical Prostatectomy?

Unlike the simple prostatectomy performed in severe cases of BPH to remove excess tissue, a radical prostatectomy (RP) involves the complete removal of the prostate gland, as well as the seminal vesicles and the lymph nodes around the prostate. To the layman, the prostate is a small organ that would seem to require relatively minor surgery to remove, but due to its location, a radical prostatectomy is actually quite formidable. The procedure may take up to four hours to perform, and because there are numerous blood vessels in the area of the prostate, the operation usually entails considerable loss of blood. Patients are encouraged to donate their blood in the weeks before the operation. Postoperative care usually involves a hospital stay from 4 to 10 days, after which the patient can go home.

There are two major forms of radical prostatectomy, based on whether a "retropubic" or "perineal" surgical technique is used. The *radical retropubic prostatectomy* is the most common form of the operation, offering the advantage of allowing for the examination of pelvic lymph nodes at the beginning of the procedure. Although diagnostic tests for identifying cancer in the lymph nodes have improved in recent years, only removal and examination of the lymph nodes can verify the presence or absence of cancer. This is important since involvement of the lymph nodes means the patient is no longer a candidate for cure using a radical prostatectomy. Once the surgeon sees the cancer has spread to the lymph nodes, the operation is most often aborted and alternative treatment options will be considered (often radiation and/or hormonal therapy).

During the operation, the patient is first anesthetized, and a long vertical incision is made in the lower abdomen, from the navel to the pubic bone. Once the incision is made, the surgeon will routinely dissect the pelvic lymph nodes for microscopic examination. The removed lymph nodes are immediately sent to a pathologist for a "frozen section" analysis, a procedure that takes about twenty minutes. The pathologist sends the results back to the surgeon. If the lymph nodes contain microscopic evidence of cancer, the pathologist will notify the surgeon, who will then decide whether to abort or proceed with the procedure.

Most urologists believe that there is little rationale for putting the patient through the operation with no chance of cure. However, some believe that if there is only minor involvement of the lymph nodes, removal of the primary tumor in the prostate may be of some advantage for the patient in reducing symptoms of the disease and extending the patient's life. Studies done at the Mayo Clinic have demonstrated that patients undergoing RP who have diploid prostate cancer fare well with hormonal therapy and that the removal of the prostate affords a significant survival advantage.

If no cancer is found by the pathologist, the operation can proceed. Access to the prostate is gained by going behind the pubic bone (hence, the name "retropubic"). The removal of the prostate is begun just above the external urethral sphincter. The prostatic urethra is divided, and the prostate is surgically removed, along with the seminal vesicles behind the bladder. The bladder neck is cut and the prostate is removed in its entirety. Then the bladder neck is pulled down and stitched to the severed end of the urethra. The larger internal sphincter must be sacrificed. During this final phase of the operation, a catheter (a ¼ inch flexible tube) is inserted into the penis, and up into the bladder to control drainage of urine. The abdominal incision is stitched up, completing the operation. The catheter remains in place for about three weeks, and is removed on a return visit to the doctor's office.

A *radical perineal prostatectomy* approaches the prostate through the perineum, the area between the scrotum and the anus. The procedure is as potentially curative as the retropubic approach, although long-term survival data is not available. The principle advantage of the perineal technique is that the postoperative recovery is much easier on the patient. However, this procedure does not allow for the dissection and examination of lymph nodes. As a consequence, most urologists reserve this technique for those with small, localized tumors, in which the likelihood of cancerous lymph nodes is very small. Some surgeons who use the perineal approach first perform an exploratory lymphadenectomy. After a few days, if the pathologist's report indicates that the lymph nodes are free of cancer, the surgeon performs the prostatectomy.

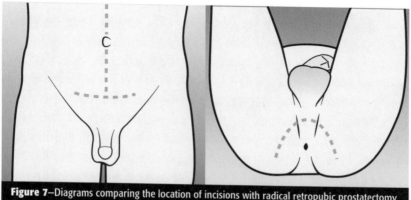

Figure 7–Diagrams comparing the location of incisions with radical retropubic prostatectomy (left) and perineal prostatectomy (right).

Which Patients are Candidates for Surgery?

Radical prostatectomy is intended as a curative treatment, and thus usually only patients with early stage prostate cancer (organ-confined disease, stages T1 and T2) are candidates for the operation. A prostatectomy is a major operation, and because of the stress and physical impact of the procedure, most surgeons discourage men older than 70 from having the operation. Because of the high risk of complications with surgery, younger men with other serious medical conditions such as heart disease are also discouraged from undergoing radical surgery.

What are the Risks of the Operation?

A prostatectomy involves some of the risks of complications that accompany any major operation. These include death associated with anesthesia, heart attack, stroke, the formation of blood clots in the legs or lungs, and infections. Fortunately, the likelihood of these complications is very small, less than 1%. Rectal damage occurs in about 1% of patients. The most common, serious complications of surgery are urinary incontinence and erectile dysfunction (see discussion below). The skill of the surgeon can significantly reduce the risk of long-term complications resulting from the procedure.

What are the Risks of Erectile Dysfunction after Radical Surgery?

Loss of sexual function is very common after surgery, since two nerve bundles associated with erection are located laterally (right / left) to the prostate gland. They closely approximate the gland at the apex (bottom). An innovative technique, pioneered by Dr. Patrick Walsh at Johns Hopkins during the early 1980's, attempts to preserve one or both of these neuro-vascular bundles (NVBs) during the radical prostatectomy. In theory, this nerve-sparing technique allows more patients to retain sexual function. However, because the technique requires shaving close to the side margins of the prostate, it is often reserved for patients whose cancer is most likely to be contained within the capsule of the prostate.

The success of the nerve-sparing procedure depends on the age and pathologic stage of the patient undergoing the operation. In the most favorable studies by the leading "artist" surgeons, men between the age of 50 and 60 have a 75% chance of retaining erectile function. Men over the age of 70 have only a 25% chance of retaining erectile function. The nerve-sparing procedure requires a high degree of surgical skill, and the results obtained by most surgeons are not as impressive as those reported by Dr. Walsh at Johns Hopkins. The National Cancer Institute has investigated the differences in results obtained by the premier surgical centers versus those obtained by less skilled practitioners utilizing the nerve-sparing technique. Researchers found that nearly all surgical patients were impotent, while 35% of patients were incontinent after treatment.

Obviously, most men have quality of life concerns, and a patient considering radical prostatectomy would be wise to ask his surgeon if he uses the nerve-sparing technique and what percentage of his patients retain erectile function. Recently developed drugs such as Viagra®, Cialis®, Levitra® and Prostatgladin E1 can be used to treat erectile dysfunction resulting from the operation, and if necessary, a penile prosthesis or other remedies may be employed. Sometimes surgery can only spare the nerves on one side of the prostate, and in the past many of these men did not retain potency. In recent years thanks to drugs like Viagra®, one side may be sufficient to allow the patient to regain some degree of potency over time.

Some other side effects of radical prostatectomy are often not candidly discussed with patients. For example, 6 to 8 months after the operation, penile shrinkage may occur because of scar tissue or the shortening of the urethra as an outcome of the procedure. For those patients who manage to retain their potency after surgery, there is no ejaculate during orgasm because the prostate gland and seminal vesicles have been removed. Orgasms experienced without ejaculate are known as dry orgasms.

When considering the pros and cons of the various treatment options, some patients are only comfortable with the idea of attempting to remove the cancer by radical surgery. This "surgical mind-set" is understandable if only because patients usually have heard more about surgery for cancer than the other treatment options, and the notion of "cutting out the cancer" appeals to some men as the simplest solution, even though the surgical data now suggests otherwise. Men who are inclined this way are strongly advised to ask their physicians if their own risk factors as determined by their test results actually make them good candidates for the procedure (see below, "What misleading arguments are used to promote surgery?").

What are the Risks of Incontinence after Surgery?

The trauma to the urine passage and bladder during radical surgery causes temporary urinary incontinence (involuntary urine leakage or dripping) in all patients. Most men regain urinary control within several weeks to several months after the operation. Others experience permanent incontinence. Loss of bladder control ranges from mild incontinence to severe incontinence, due to permanent damage done to the urethral sphincter. Severe incontinence occurs in about 5% of patients. In these cases, exercises, medications or the surgical placement of an artificial sphincter may be used to restore urinary control to the patient.

There are generally three types of incontinence: stress incontinence, overflow incontinence, and urgency incontinence. Men with stress incontinence, the most common type after surgery, leak urine when they cough, laugh, get up or turn quickly, or lift heavy objects. Men with overflow incontinence take a long time to urinate and have a weak or dribbling stream. Men with urgency incontinence experience a sudden need to pass urine.

There is a wide variation in the medical literature as far as the likelihood that patients will experience incontinence after surgery. The numbers may vary anywhere from 5% to 65%. This discrepancy is primarily due to the fact that doctors use different definitions to describe incontinence. If a patient has only slight leakage (for example, only one diaper daily), some doctors report that the patient is not incontinent, while other doctors consider a patient with any urine leakage to be incontinent. A realistic estimate of the likelihood of incontinence would probably be about 25% of patients with the best surgical care.

Why is Hormonal Therapy sometimes used Before Surgery?

Hormonal therapy, also known as Androgen Ablation Therapy (ADT), can shrink a man's prostate up to 50%. Some surgeons recommend the use of hormonal therapy for several months prior to surgery. The rationale is that reducing the size of the prostate will make it easier to remove. While there is no definitive proof that hormonal downsizing will increase the likelihood of cure with surgery, it remains a valid option for some patients. Many surgeons discourage hormones since they believe that there is more capsular scarring, making it especially difficult to excise the gland or spare the nerve bundles. Others use hormones as a temporary regimen, allowing the patient more time to explore his treatment options without concern about cancer progression.

What are the Treatment Options If Surgery Fails?

In men who show a measurable PSA after surgery (often defined as a PSA of 0.2 or higher), the likelihood is that some cancer was left at the margins of the prostate or that some cancer may have spread to other areas of the body, even though it may not be detected by lymph node dissection or by bone scans. In these cases, further surgery is not advisable.

A second attempt at a cure with another type of treatment is called "salvage therapy," because it attempts to salvage a cure after an initial treatment failure. The common forms of salvage therapy for patients who are at risk for failure after surgery are radiation therapy and hormonal therapy. Many patients are clinically understaged and are found to have *positive surgical margins* (cancer beyond the gland and outside the surgical field), or to have extracapsular extension or seminal vesicle involvement either at the time of surgery or pathologically. Some of these patients may opt for watchful waiting to see if their PSA starts rising before they decide to embark on another course of therapy.

Instead of waiting for the PSA to signal a recurrence of cancer, some urologists encourage patients in this category to begin a course of radiation therapy in the hope of avoiding problems later. This is referred to as *adjuvant radiation therapy*. Radiation is delivered to the prostatic region in the hope that it will destroy any cancer that may remain there. External radiation following surgery has been shown to reduce the risk of biochemical relapse (rising PSA) by approximately 30% (as evidenced by the fact that about 30% of men show an undetectable PSA after salvage radiation). There are many patients whose cancers are resistant to radiation or have already metastasized, and therefore, are not likely to benefit from radiation as a salvage treatment. To minimize the risk of complications, doctors usually allow surgical patients to recover for 3 to 6 months before starting radiation therapy.

External radiation is the most common salvage treatment for presumed local failure after surgery, while hormonal therapy is most often prescribed in cases of distant failure and evidence of metastatic disease. Some doctors favor using hormonal therapy after surgery as soon as there is any evidence of recurrence. The rationale is that hormones may slow the progress of the disease for some time. The idea of a hormonal cure is doubtful, but hormones do interrupt the spread of the disease temporarily. For some men, this knowledge may be enough to prompt them to try some form of hormonal intervention early on. Other patients may prefer to wait. Recent data, however, suggests that early hormonal intervention is superior to delayed treatment.

Depending on the particular hormone or combination of hormones that are prescribed, many men experience some side effects such as erectile dysfunction, loss of sexual desire (libido), breast enlargement, hot flashes, nausea, diarrhea, liver enzyme elevation, muscle weakness, joint aches or pains, and bone fragility (loss of bone integrity). Depending on the type of hormone prescribed, there are also a number of medications and treatment options which should be used to minimize or ameliorate these side effects.

Patients who opt for watchful waiting after local failure with surgery must be monitored very carefully. Waiting means being prepared to treat specific symptoms of the disease with radiation and/or hormonal therapies if and when it becomes necessary to do so. As will be discussed in more detail later, hormones sooner or later will cease to be effective, though this can take many years for some men. When this occurs, the cancer is referred to as hormone refractory or hormone resistant. When hormonal therapy fails to stop the prostate cancer from spreading, the cancer may behave aggressively, with progression being imminent. In this situation, chemotherapy (cytotoxic systemic agents) may be considered (see Chapter Eight: Treating Metastatic Disease).

Why is Surgery No Longer the Treatment of Choice for Most Patients?

Historically, radical prostatectomy was for many years the primary treatment for early stage prostate cancer and most urologists regarded it as the "gold standard" treatment (and most still hang on to that belief despite data to the contrary). Since urologists are the specialists who see most prostate cancer patients after diagnosis, it is not surprising that they recommend their specialty and that in the past most patients chose the surgical option. That situation has changed in recent years with advances in alternative, non-surgical treatments such as radiation therapy. With more men being diagnosed earlier thanks to PSA screening and patients doing more research prior to embarking on a treatment course, the number of radical prostatectomies has fallen dramatically since the early 1990s. That trend is likely to continue as more patients opt for non-surgical treatments with comparable or superior cure rates and a lower risk of complications.

What Cure Rates have been Reported by the Premier Surgeons?

When comparing radical surgery with other treatment options in the PSA era, findings have been consistent when grouping patients in low, intermediate and high risk categories. With a follow-up of ten years or longer, prostatectomy appears to be effective in 80% to 90% of patients, as reported by teams from the leading specialty centers, but this success rate applies only to patients with low risk, favorable tumors (PSA < 10, Gleason score ≤ 6, clinical stage T2a or less).

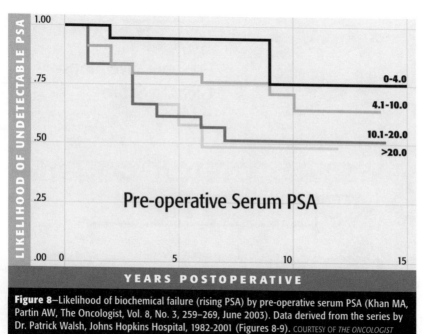

Figure 8—Likelihood of biochemical failure (rising PSA) by pre-operative serum PSA (Khan MA, Partin AW, The Oncologist, Vol. 8, No. 3, 259–269, June 2003). Data derived from the series by Dr. Patrick Walsh, Johns Hopkins Hospital, 1982-2001 (Figures 8-9). COURTESY OF *THE ONCOLOGIST*

With intermediate and high risk patients (PSA greater than 10, Gleason 7 to 10, clinical state equal to or greater than T2b), the data shows that these patients have a high risk for biochemical failure after radical prostatectomy. Indeed, it is with the higher risk groups that the results obtained with surgery have deteriorated to the point of being woefully unacceptable. The lack of any plateau in the disease-free survival curves of surgery patients with a pre-treatment PSA above 10 and/or a Gleason score of 7 or higher is especially striking coming from a leading institution like Johns Hopkins (see Figures 8-9). Note that these researchers defined biochemical disease-free survival after surgery as having an undetectable PSA.

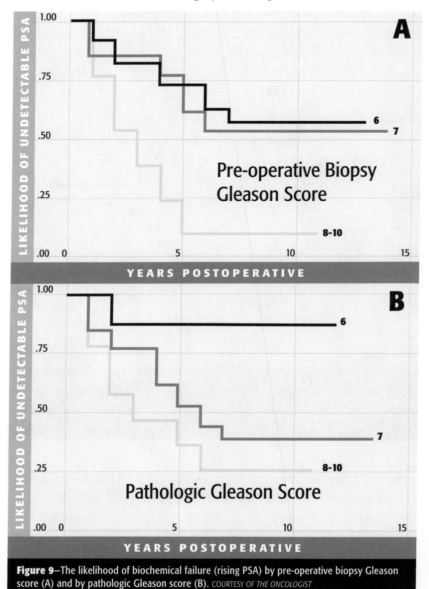

Figure 9–The likelihood of biochemical failure (rising PSA) by pre-operative biopsy Gleason score (A) and by pathologic Gleason score (B). COURTESY OF *THE ONCOLOGIST*

What Misleading Arguments are used to Promote Surgery?

While legitimate arguments can be made for and against each type of treatment, a number of misleading arguments are often made in favor of the use of surgery over radiation. The common sense notion of "cutting the cancer out" is used to imply that a radical prostatectomy is the most effective therapy. But the fact is that 50% or more of patients with intermediate or high risk cancers will fail after surgery.

Another argument often used to promote surgery over radiation is the assertion that if a patient undergoes radiation and it fails, then surgery as a salvage treatment will not be an option. In fact, this is not the case. Many experienced surgeons will perform a prostatectomy at this point, albeit the operation is more difficult, as tissue that has been irradiated becomes more fragile. Depending on the institution reporting, between 10% and 50% of these patients can be cured by a salvage prostatectomy. Complications such as incontinence and erectile dysfunction increase somewhat, and the surgeons appear to be far more willing to disclose these complications which they can attribute to the radiation. Complication rates are relatively high according to a National Cancer Institute investigation of patients treated primarily with radical surgery (without receiving radiation), although the surgeons appear to be less forthcoming in this regard.

Treatment options for patients who have failed radiation are actually quite numerous. In addition to a salvage prostatectomy, they may include salvage brachytherapy, Intensity Modulated Radiation Therapy and brachytherapy (combined), and cryosurgery (all of which are discussed in greater detail below). It is the flip side of the coin that is actually more troublesome – the patient who has had surgery and fails. At this point, it is often unclear whether the PSA is rising due to local recurrence, or distant relapse (which may be microscopic and not detected by bone scans, CT scans, MRI, etc.) or both. In this situation, only salvage radiation is an option for potential cure, and recent studies demonstrate that only 10% to 30% of patients can be successfully salvaged (rescued).

CHAPTER SIX

RADIATION THERAPY

What is Radiation and How Does It Work?

X-ray radiation is a form of energy similar to visible light. When directed at the body, x-rays penetrate tissue and are gradually absorbed. Some of the radiation is absorbed by cells and damages the DNA that normally allows cells to function and reproduce. Cancer cells are somewhat more sensitive to radiation than are healthy cells, and therefore, the radiation used to destroy cancer cells is less likely to damage normal tissues, which are tenacious. However, this difference in sensitivity is generally small and the dose of radiation required to destroy prostate cancer cells is high enough that there is some risk of damage to healthy tissue in the nearby rectum or bladder.

The strategy with radiation therapy over the years has been to deliver higher and higher doses more and more accurately to the targeted cancer, while sparing healthy adjacent tissue in order to avoid rectal and urinary complications. Since the 1950s, external radiation therapy has been a common technique used for the treatment of many kinds of cancers. It is a standard treatment for prostate cancer that is clinically confined to the prostate and surrounding tissues (stages T1, T2, and T3). It may also be prescribed for patients with stage N+ disease, prostate cancer that has spread to the pelvic lymph nodes. Patients with advanced prostate cancer may also be treated with external radiation as a palliative (non-curative) therapy to reduce the size of the tumor and alleviate symptoms.

What is External Beam Radiation Therapy?

With the conventional approach known as external beam radiation therapy (EBRT), high energy X-rays are targeted directly to the region of the prostate to kill or incapacitate any cancer cells in the area. The machine most widely used today to administer EBRT is the linear accelerator, which uses electrical principles (electrons) to generate photon radiation. The linear accelerator has largely replaced an older generation of machines that utilized radioactive cobalt and were not as accurate.

Radiation is given to the patient in small daily doses, usually five days a week over a course of 7 to 8 weeks. Delivering small, incremental doses over time decreases the chance of damaging healthy tissue. Radiation is completely painless and cannot be felt by the patient. Typically, a single treatment can be carried out in several minutes. Radiation is measured by a unit called the Gray (Gy), roughly analogous to a Watt of light. Radiotherapists often describe radiation dose rates in terms of centigray (cGy), or 100 Gray units (what used to be called a "rad"). A typical daily dose of external radiation may range from about 180 to 200 centigray.

Preparation for radiation therapy is a rigorously complex process that involves exact determination of the region to receive treatment and the appropriate dose of radiation. Radiation treatments are precisely designed for each patient, because each man's prostate and surrounding organs are unique in size and shape. A planning session is carried out with the patient several days before treatments begin. In order to keep the patient in the same position for each daily treatment, he may be fitted to a custom-made plastic mold. Once the patient's body is properly aligned, fluoroscopic and ultrasound imaging techniques are used to visualize the prostate and nearby organs. The position of these critical structures will determine where the radiation beams should be directed and also the shape of the beams. During treatment, beams from several directions converge to form a high-dose target zone, which includes the prostate and a margin of tissue surrounding the gland. The radiation can be focused on the target area while minimizing the risk of over-radiating the rectum and bladder.

What are the Risks of Side Effects with External Radiation?

As with radical prostatectomy, there are possible side effects with external beam radiation therapy. Common side effects are fatigue, urinary urgency, frequency and burning on urination, and rectal irritation. The majority of these symptoms will disappear after treatment is concluded, but in some cases damage to the bladder or, less frequently, to the rectum results in chronic complications. These include urethral and bladder inflammation and the need to urinate more frequently (urethritis, cystitis), and intermittent periods of rectal bleeding or rectal urgency that may continue for years afterwards. Severe bladder or rectal injury is very rare. Although most men retain erectile function after the conclusion of radiation therapy, as many as half of the men who undergo conventional EBRT will eventually develop erectile dysfunction.

The skill of the radiotherapist administering treatments can significantly reduce the risk of complications, as can the use of more advanced technology. Conventional EBRT has largely been replaced in this country by more sophisticated techniques for delivering radiation. As discussed below, 3-D Conformal Radiation, Intensity Modulated Radiation Therapy, and brachytherapy have shown superior results both for curing the cancer and reducing the likelihood of complications.

What is 3D-Conformal Radiation Therapy?

In the past, some researchers suggested that radiation therapy might only halt progression of the disease for a number of years, after which the cancer would recur. But many radiotherapists argued that this was only the case if the radiation beam was imprecisely directed during treatment and thus failed to deliver a sufficient cancer-killing dose. Until the mid-1980's, the maximum dose that could be safely administered to the prostate was thought to be 7000 centigray. Higher doses at that time were associated with an unacceptably high risk of complications. With the improved technologies in use today, doses of 7000 to 8000 centigray are common with the technique known as 3D-Conformal Radiation (3DCRT), which has greatly reduced the risk of complications.

Since the mid-1980's, three-dimensional computerized imaging techniques have vastly improved the accuracy of external radiation and allowed for the safe delivery of increased doses. Guided by these technological innovations, the radiotherapist molds blocks of lead alloy to conform precisely to the outline of the tumor. In order to shield healthy tissues and organs that are to be avoided, the blocks are clamped to the end of the linear accelerator, and by this means, the radiation treatment is precisely tailored for each individual patient.

Five and ten year results with 3D-Conformal Radiation Therapy have been very favorable. Because of the increased accuracy, side effects of conformal radiation are less common than with the traditional application of external beam radiation therapy. In addition, the increased dose delivered by 3DCRT has increased cure rates to a point comparable to those achieved with surgery. Yet even this relatively advanced technique for delivering external radiation has been surpassed by cutting edge modalities such as Intensity Modulated Radiation Therapy and brachytherapy.

Does Dose Matter?

The results of a Memorial Sloan-Kettering study that compared 5-year biochemical disease-free survival among patient risk groups receiving low dose (6480 to 7020 cGy) versus high dose (7560 to 8640 cGy). Note that higher doses showed a significant advantage for all risk groups (Zelefsky, et al).

RISK GROUP	LOW DOSE	HIGH DOSE
Low	77%	90%
Intermediate	50%	70%
High	21%	47%

What is Intensity Modulated Radiation Therapy?

Intensity Modulated Radiation Therapy (IMRT) is currently the state of the art when it comes to external radiation therapy, taking 3D-CRT to an even higher level of precision and control (See Color Inset Images 3-A, 3-B). With IMRT, the single beam of radiation is replaced by thousands of "beamlets" or "micro-beams," each with its own intensity and energy level as directed by the radiotherapist. A unique treatment blueprint is mapped out in advance for each patient. With computer planning and three-dimensional imaging techniques, the physician is able to more accurately deliver radiation to satisfy pre-defined dose specifications to the tumor while avoiding nearby healthy tissue. Thus, the risk of damaging the bowel, bladder, rectum and other organs is significantly reduced. At the same time, the cancer-killing dose of radiation is maximized on the designated target.

How is IMRT Planned and Performed?

With IMRT, each treatment volume is considered on a voxel by voxel basis (with a voxel being a cubic millimeter of space) and each voxel may receive a different dose. This is like treating an area the size of a tip of a pen. Once the "target" has been designated, a planning phase referred to as "inverse treatment planning" generates beam profiles with varying intensities across the treatment field. The intensity profile of each beamlet is adjusted to satisfy the predefined dose specifications to the tumor as well as to the normal tissues. A computer, using mathematical optimization algorithms, then runs the optimization program, which selects the best combination of directions and beam intensities to obtain the ideal optimized plan. The program consists of literally thousands of discreet angles and doses.

To accomplish the planning phase, extremely sophisticated computerized software is utilized and plans are generated in a time frame measured in hours. This task might take a world class physicist years to accomplish. Since we are generating high-energy beamlets at specific cubic millimeter targets, immobilization of the patient is imperative. For this reason, a number of checks and balances are put into place. For example, for each patient, a customized "alpha-cradle" (similar to a body cast or mold) is designed for immobilization of the lower body in the supine position.

Once the patient's treatment profile has been digitally reconstructed, and a specific program or "blueprint" for that patient is developed, verification of the IMRT treatment is performed by utilizing amorphous silicone diode imaging, which is referred to as "Portal Vision." This silicon diode has unprecedented resolution and image acquisition, so that the doctor can watch the treatment in "real time," or review this program at the workstation at a later time. The actual delivery of the radiation is a dynamic process and is accomplished through the use of multi-leaf collimators. These devices essentially allow us to "sculpt" the beams in order to deliver the precise dose required (see Color Inset Images 3-B, 3-C, 3-E, 3-F, 3-G, 3-H, 3-I).

Prior to each treatment, an ultrasound-based machine known as a *B-Mode Acquisition and Targeting Transducer* (BAT) is employed to make sure that the prostate and the tumor are in the exact same location each day for each beam application which was initially prescribed (as these targets are dynamic and may move from one treatment day to the next). The BAT interfaces with the main computer and insures that the optimized plan is indeed being carried out. This is crucial since fluid levels may vary in the bladder, while air and contents within the rectum can also change daily.

Even the simple motion of breathing can shift the position of the prostate, which is tracked and corrected for by a special "Respiratory Gating" device. Daily localization of the target is essential to optimize therapeutic effects since both patient and organ movement may occur. It should be noted that all the techniques described—Portal Vision, BAT transducer, Respiratory Gating—are non-invasive. These routines are implemented with comprehensive checklists that are crucial to ensure accurate targeting on a daily

IMRT Analysis Tools

BAT (B-Mode Acquisition and Targeting System)
Ultrasound-based daily verification of target organ position

Portal Vision
Amorphous silicon imaging technology which allows for real time on-line verification of the patient's exact treatment position

Respiratory Gating
Advanced video tracking technology which allows for realtime monitoring and correction of physiologic motion of prostate which may occur as a result of patient breathing

basis. Even one omission in the checklist can mean the difference between striking the target or landing outside the target with inappropriate doses.

Most patients are treated Monday through Friday for approximately four to five weeks. They are seen daily by the radiation technologists and at least once a week by a nurse as well as the doctor. After completion of the IMRT, many patients return in three to six weeks for brachytherapy, if their risk factors mandate a combined approach.

How does IMRT Compare to 3D-CRT?

While IMRT is not yet widely used outside of major medical centers, recent studies comparing IMRT to 3D-CRT have demonstrated a very significant advantage for IMRT with respect to both success rates and reduction of side effects. One study from Memorial Sloan-Kettering showed IMRT increased the success rate in shrinking tumors from 43% to 96%, while decreasing complications from 10% to 2%. Our IMRT team and others are reporting similar findings. As we will see in the pages ahead, IMRT offers even greater advantages when it is combined with brachytherapy, especially with intermediate and high risk patients. It should also be noted that IMRT is not considered an experimental procedure, but is rather the culmination of earlier external radiation delivery systems. IMRT is both FDA and Medicare approved, and its effectiveness has already been demonstrated by many scientific studies.

Which Patients are Eligible for External Radiation Therapy?

Because external radiation (EBRT, 3D-CRT, and IMRT) is non-invasive and does not require an operation or anesthesia, most men can safely tolerate this form of therapy. The likelihood of cure is greatest with low risk patients (clinical stage T1, non-palpable tumors, less than 50% core involvement found in the biopsy specimens, a Gleason score $\leq$ 6, serum PSA $\leq$ 10, and a non-elevated PAP). Intermediate and high risk patients can also be effectively treated with external radiation, but more favorable results for these patients are now being achieved when external radiation is combined with brachytherapy.

Even patients having locally advanced disease with regional lymph node involvement have enjoyed long disease-free intervals and even a cure. Patients with metastatic disease beyond the regional lymph nodes cannot be cured with radiation; however, they may be treated with radiation if the cancer in the region of the prostate is causing symptomatic urinary or rectal problems. Patients with bone metastases may also receive radiation to relieve pain.

What is Brachytherapy?

Brachytherapy, also called *interstitial implantation therapy,* involves the placement of tiny radioactive seeds or pellets directly into the prostate gland. The radioactive seeds can either be inserted temporarily, or can remain permanently in place within the prostate. They provide a high dose of radiation that is concentrated in the prostate. Permanent seeds pose no health threat to the patient, as they decay within 6 months to a year, and thereafter, they become inert.

Brachytherapy has a fairly long history. As early as 1917, a crude form of seed implantation using radium needles was performed at what is now Memorial Sloan-Kettering Cancer Center. The chief of urology at that time, Dr. Barringer, was so enthusiastic about the procedure that he concluded his report in the *Journal of the American Medical Association,* "...because of the initial success of radium treatment, I now take the stand that no patient with prostate cancer should be operated on." In fact, the technology had not yet been developed that would make the procedure effective. The 1980's saw renewed interest in seed implants because the development of ultrasound imaging, CT scans and fluoroscopic techniques allowed for precise planning and monitoring of where the seeds should be placed. Since that time, brachytherapy has become a standard, mainstream treatment for prostate cancer that is widely available throughout the U.S.

As with external radiation therapy, a number of technical refinements in the seed implant procedure have led to improved results and increasing popularity. In the old days (as recently as the 1970's), seed implants required major abdominal surgery. Seeds of radioactive isotopes were manually implanted into the prostate using needles, but the procedure was essentially carried out blind and achieved poor results because of a lack of precision in placing the seeds. Poor placement led to "cold" spots within the prostate gland that did not receive a sufficient dose of radiation to destroy the cancer.

In more recent years, a minimally invasive technique has been devised for implanting the seeds in the prostate without open surgery (known as "transperineal implantation"). Guided by ultrasound and fluoroscopy, the seeds are dispensed through tiny hollow needles which are inserted through the perineum (the area between the scrotum and anus). A template or grid is used to precisely guide the placement of the needles. Ultrasound allows for real time imaging and dynamic visualization. As the technology has evolved with color-flow Doppler ultrasound, a more precise, three-dimensional image of the prostate can be generated, and the seeds can be more accurately placed, where they will do the most good (See Color Inset Images 2-A, 2-B, 2-C, 2-D, 2-E, 2F). As with external radiation therapy, the strategy has been to target and destroy the cancer with minimal exposure to surrounding healthy tissue and organs. The computerized guidance system helps determine where the seeds should go, how deeply they should be inserted, and how strong their radiation should be.

Brachytherapy with ultrasound and fluoroscopic guidance has a number of advantages over conventional external beam radiation therapy. The standard dose of radiation used with EBRT is approximately 7000 cGy, calculated to be the highest dose which is safe and well tolerated by the patient. By contrast, seed implants are placed internally to deliver radiation directly to the prostate while sparing surrounding organs. As a consequence, higher doses of radiation (exceeding 12,000 cGy) can be administered to the area of the prostate, while tumorous sites often receive doses in excess of 20,000 cGy. In addition, the radiation delivered by seeds is continuous over the time they are active, working around the clock to kill the cancer. By contrast, all other forms of radiation, including HDR

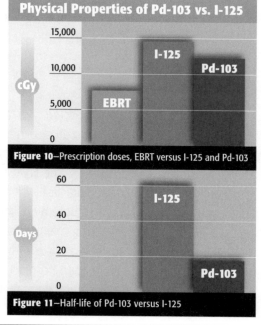

Figure 10—Prescription doses, EBRT versus I-125 and Pd-103

Figure 11—Half-life of Pd-103 versus I-125

(see below) are fractionated, which means the radiation is administered only in intermittent doses.

A number of radiation sources have been used for interstitial implantation. The most commonly used permanent implants are encapsulated isotopes of either Palladium-103 or Iodine-125. Pd-103 has a significantly shorter half-life (the period of time until its output of radiation is halved) and a greater initial radiation dose than I-125 (see Figures 10-11). With palladium, the radiation dosage is delivered in three to four months compared to up to one year with iodine. Because the radiation is active for a shorter period with palladium, temporary side effects such as urinary distress are shorter in duration.

What is High Does Rate (HDR) Brachytherapy?

High Dose Rate brachytherapy refers to temporary implants that utilize Iridium-192. This form of therapy is not new. It was first utilized in 1964 at Memorial Sloan-Kettering Cancer Center and has remained essentially unchanged since that time, with the exception of the current use of microprocessors and advanced imaging techniques.

The Iridium-192 isotope is encased inside a hollow plastic catheter less than 2 millimeters in diameter. Typically guided by ultrasound, these implants are inserted into the prostate and then removed, with two to four separate procedures spread over two to three days. HDR sources deliver much higher doses of radiation in a much shorter period of time than permanent implants.

Some limited studies have reported cure rates with the temporary HDR procedure that are comparable to those achieved by permanent implants. There is, however, far less data regarding outcomes and side effects when compared to permanent implants. The HDR approach is not widely used for reasons of convenience and practicality. If performed in one setting, the patient must remain in a semi-lithotomy position (legs pulled up) for upwards of 72 hours, with needles remaining in the prostate throughout this duration. Like external radiation, HDR is a form of fractionated radiation. Temporary implants usually require hospitalization and repeated implant procedures as opposed to the single permanent implant technique which can be done essentially on an out-patient basis. There may also be a greater risk of complications with HDR because of the extremely penetrating, high dose of radiation delivered by the Iridium-192 isotope (1000 to 2000 cGy in a matter of minutes). The discussion that follows will be devoted to permanent Pd-103 and I-125 implantation.

MODALITY	TYPICAL DOSE	DELIVERY
3D-CRT	7000–8000 cGy	Fractionated
IMRT	7000–9000 cGy	Fractionated
Protons/Neutrons	7000–8000 cGy	Fractionated
Pd-103/I-125 Brachytherapy (Monotherapy)	12,500/14,400 cGy	Continuous
HDR Ir-192 (Monotherapy)	?	Fractionated
3D-CRT/IMRT and Pd-103/I-125	4000–5000 cGy 8000–12,000 cGy	Fractionated Continuous
EBRT and HDR Ir-192 and Pd-103/I-125	4000–5000 cGy 1500–2500 cGy	Fractionated Fractionated

A Comparison of Radiotherapy Modalities for Treatment of Localized (loco-regional) Prostate Cancer

How are Permanent Seed Implants Planned and Performed?

At our institution, patients routinely undergo a pre-treatment staging and planning color-flow Doppler ultrasound. That test, coupled with other staging studies (e.g. EMRI, MRSI, Prostascint™ and CT Fusion) will allow us to visualize various physical aspects of the gland, such as its size, shape, and contour. These tests also provide detailed information about the volume and location of the tumor (or tumors). With that information, we are able to determine exactly where the seeds should be placed. Additionally, this pre-treatment analysis may tell us if the public bones are going pose any sort of obstacle when we perform the procedure. This is known as pubic arch interference, which we can usually circumvent by positioning the patient more advantageously. Later, in the operating room, the original plan may be modified if the gland position or contour changes.

Prior to the implant procedure, I ask my patients not to eat after midnight the night before and the morning of the implant. A patient is admitted to the hospital as an outpatient for 23-hour observation. After admission, he is routinely given a prophylactic antibiotic. The patient is then brought into a surgical suite, or a dedicated brachytherapy suite, and there undergoes an antiseptic skin cleansing. That is usually a Betadine solution applied to the perineal region. We also provide him with pre-implant bowel cleansing instructions and are ready to proceed with the procedure after administering a local anesthetic in most cases (epidural or spinal anesthesia).

The procedure is done with the patient lying on his back, with his legs pulled up in what is called the *extended lithotomy position.* His legs are completely limp since a local anesthesia has been delivered. His feet are placed in comfortable booties and held in stirrups. Considerable time is spent ensuring that the patient is in the proper position and that the prostate is in the exact position that it was when the pre-planning volumetric analysis was performed. This is not always possible, and in such cases, necessary adjustments are made. Then the implant procedure is performed using both ultrasound and fluoroscopic guidance.

The isotopes used for brachytherapy don't deliver much radiation at a distance of a centimeter or centimeter and a half away from the gland, which is, for example, where the rectum and the bladder reside. The seeds are placed precisely at the site of the cancer within a margin of approximately 1 to 5 millimeters outside the prostate capsule. By this means, we can often deliver two to five times the dose with brachytherapy that we can with any other kind of radiation.

The dose rate is in the range of 20 cGy per hour with Palladium-103 compared to 5 to 10 cGy per hour with Iodine-125. A total dose of 12,500 cGy is typically delivered with Palladium-103 to full decay, while 14,500 cGy is typically delivered with Iodine-125. If I am supplementing the seed implant by preceding it with IMRT, then I have to reduce the dose of the implant. With this combined or integrated approach, patients typically receive 4100 cGy of external radiation to a limited pelvic field, followed approximately three to six weeks later by a Palladium-103 "boost." When combined with IMRT, the prescribed minimum Pd-103 dose to the prostate is 8000 to 9000 cGy.

Seed implants are performed in a specially designed operating room (OR) where computers are accessible for intra-operative modifications. A well-trained OR staff is utilized for the procedure. Local anesthesia (spinal versus epidural) is preferred. The advantage of a local anesthetic is that the patient feels little or no discomfort upon awakening, including that of a catheter, which is put into place during the implant procedure. Anti-inflammatory medications and antibiotics are routinely administered during and after the procedure (intraoperative and postoperative).

We maintain computers in the operating room in the event that the contour of the prostate gland changes. This may happen because for the first time we are looking at the prostate in a relaxed position without the pelvic muscles surrounding it being very tense. Because the patient has undergone a local anesthetic, he cannot tense up around the ultrasound probe which is placed in the rectum. If there are substantial contour changes, we have the ability to make intraoperative modifications of the plan as necessary.

The actual procedure, that is, the placement of the needles and insertion of the seeds, rarely takes longer than twenty-five minutes. The set-up time and preparation of the patient may take longer, and therefore, I generally book an hour and a half in the OR, because the patient has to be placed in the proper position and prepped for the procedure. It's very important to have the patient in a position that is identical to that of his pre-planning study so as not to depart from the initial plan. When performing the procedure, special crisscross anchoring needles are used to maximally immobilize the prostate gland. These two crisscross needles are inserted transperineally, obliquely into the prostate, using finger and fluoroscopic guidance. These needles are left in place during the procedure to anchor the prostate in place.

Seeds are commonly placed in extracapsular positions to further target the tumor, which may be microscopically escaping from the gland. The technique of placing seeds 1 to 5 millimeters outside the gland also allows for reduction of the urethral dose. This is important since the main side effect of brachytherapy is temporary urethritis. Additionally, this technique allows for treating patients who have had prior TURPS with a far reduced incontinence rate.

After the procedure, the patient is transferred to a private room and monitored closely throughout his stay. Although many brachytherapists discharge their patients soon after the implant is complete, I prefer to keep the patient overnight. The indwelling catheter is left in place for a minimum of 12 hours and dislodges any tissue, clots or debris that could present future problems (urinary blockage). The catheter is removed only when upon inspection the urine is perfectly clear. Usually, I keep the catheters in until three o'clock in the morning. That saves a lot of grief for the patient and for me by eliminating those calls that I might receive at 2:00 A.M. when the patient potentially has some blockage. By keeping the catheter in and irrigating the bladder, we have fewer problems.

For the most part, patients have a very easy time with seed implants. The most common question asked after the procedure is, "When are you going to start?" Many are still waiting for the procedure to begin when they realize it has already taken place. Patients rarely complain of specific pains in the perineal region, that area where the seeds are implanted between the scrotal sac and the anus. The only discomfort that a patient may have is more likely to be a consequence of the catheter. That may be felt more than the tiny needles which are utilized to insert the seeds.

The patient is discharged the morning following the procedure, usually in excellent spirits and ready to return home whether far away or locally. Prior to his leaving our center, special stereo-shift x-rays and helical CT scans are taken to count seeds and to ensure there are no potential complications (for example, absess formation or hematomas from bleeding, though these are uncommon). Patients will then return for a comprehensive evaluation at approximately three months, six months, and annually thereafter.

Which Patients are Eligible for Brachytherapy?

Most patients can safely tolerate the implant procedure as it is minimally invasive and requires only light anesthesia. Men with a history of heart disease or stroke are usually given a thorough medical evaluation, including a cardiac stress test, before proceeding with seed implantation.

If you are a candidate for surgery, you are almost surely also a candidate for seed implants, as both treatments are most effective with early stage cancers. In addition, many men who would not be candidates for surgery–those patients over the age of 70, or those men with other health conditions that rule out major surgery–may qualify as candidates for seeding, which is obviously a much less invasive procedure than radical prostatectomy.

The most important factor in determining a patient's eligibility for seeding is how far the cancer has spread. If the cancer is localized, that is, confined to the prostate gland, then it is more likely to be curable, with either surgery or seeding. Once the cancer has spread beyond the prostate capsule, it is not curable by implantation alone, because the seed implants do not radiate enough area around the prostate to destroy any cancer that may have spread beyond the prostate capsule. These patients are similarly not candidates for radical prostatectomy.

Patients with stage T1 are most likely to have cancer that is confined to the prostate, and therefore, curable with seed implantation alone. Patients with locally advanced disease may be treated either with external radiation or with a combination of seed implants and external radiation (preferably IMRT). These patients include those with one or more of the following risk factors: stage equal to or greater than T2b, a Gleason score greater than or equal to 7, a PSA greater than 10, an elevated PAP, or radiographic evidence of extracapsular extension (as indicated by color-flow Doppler ultrasound or endorectal EMRI).

Seed implants should only be considered by patients who are young enough and healthy enough to live long enough to benefit from being cured. Excellent candidates are men from their forties to their seventies, with localized prostate cancer. As mentioned earlier, some men in their eighties who are in good health may also benefit from implantation, and an increasing number of men in their thirties are now being treated with these methods.

Patients who have had a portion of their prostate removed with a previous TURP may be at increased risk for urinary incontinence after seeding. Patients with enlarged prostates and those men who have difficulty with urination prior to treatment may have more severe urinary problems after implantation. Treatment is typically restricted to men with prostates less than 60 cubic centimeters volume. For patients with enlarged prostates, two or three months of hormonal therapy before implantation may be prescribed in order to shrink the gland.

When is Hormonal Therapy Used Prior to Brachytherapy?

Hormonal treatment is typically optional for patients having intermediate risk features but encouraged for patients having high risk features. With the low-risk or mildly aggressive cancers, unless the size of the gland is markedly large, we don't normally give the conventional hormonal therapy (combined hormonal blockade using an anti-androgen and an LHRH agonist), since this form of therapy may result in untoward side effects such as impotence, hot flashes and potential weakness. We often prescribe a milder, modified version of hormones (e.g. oral anti-androgens), something that is just enough to arrest the cancer and allow the patient to make a more relaxed decision about treatment, without the rush or urgency that are often associated with it (see Chapter Eight: Treating Metastatic Disease).

Why are More Patients Choosing to Combine Seed Implants with IMRT?

Over the past decade I have seen the pendulum swing dramatically from patients in the past who strongly desired to undergo seed implantations alone to more recent patients who desire the combination method of IMRT and brachytherapy. This trend is probably due to a number of factors. These days many patients do extensive research and find that there is always a real risk of having extracapsular disease extension, which is more effectively treated by integrating seed implants with IMRT (or 3D-CRT). Many patients now understand that with IMRT they are afforded the added security of covering possible extracapsular extension while experiencing little to no additional side effects.

What are the Possible Side Effects of Seed Implantation?

Seed implantation involves significantly less risk of long-term complications compared with surgery or conventional EBRT. Side effects with implants are usually mild and reversible. The most common organ system involved with temporary side effects from seed implants is the urinary tract, and this is because the prostate is nestled beneath the bladder and has the urethra running through it. Following implantation, most patients experience increased urinary frequency and urgency, a weakened stream, and occasionally, urinary burning. Fortunately, these symptoms are temporary and resolve as the radioactivity of the seeds dissipates over time.

With palladium implants, the 17-day half-life typically causes about two and a half to four months of some type of urinary symptomology. With the 60-day half-life of iodine implants, urinary symptoms may persist for ten to twelve months. During this period, we do our best to micromanage these urinary symptoms with a variety of medications. The symptoms are in no way debilitating, but rather more of a nuisance, and patients are encouraged to continue their normal level of activity.

While side effects with implantation are usually temporary, there is some risk of more serious, permanent complications, including urinary incontinence (in less than 1% of patients) and erectile dysfunction. When they do occur, such side effects usually appear 6 to 24 months after treatment. As mentioned, patients who have previously undergone TURPs are at higher risk for developing incontinence. Incontinence is a very rare complication associated with implantation therapy in general for patients without TURPs—less than 1% in virtually all studies. But patients with prior TURPs are more likely to develop urinary incontinence, up to 50% according to some researchers. However, brachytherapists who modify their implants and make adjustments for patients with TURPs have reported incontinence in less than 3% of patients (see below, "How are implants modified for patients with prior TURPs?").

Another potential side effect with seeds is irritation to the rectum, although this is uncommon. In my experience with the procedure, I don't have one patient who has had to have a colostomy or who has a persistent rectal ulceration; nor do I have any patients who required urinary diversion because of damage to the urethra. It appears that while the urethra tends to play an important role with seeding in terms of the side effect profile, it generally is able to withstand the dose, and once the seeds decay, the side effects disappear.

What is the Risk of Erectile Dysfunction after seed Implantation?

Generally speaking, patients having prostate brachytherapy will have erectile dysfunction in about 15% to 20% of cases, although some institutions are reporting higher rates of incidence. Brachytherapy does not appear to produce the steady decline of potency that we have seen with full course external beam radiation through the years. Rather, I have noted not only a leveling off of the potency rate over time after implantation, but even a gradual improvement over time. Essentially, where you are at two to three years after treatment is where you will likely be as far as erectile function, taking into account that patients are getting older and may be taking hypertensive medications, diabetic medications or have other medical problems which could interfere with erectile function over time. Smoking and obesity are also significant causal factors for erectile dysfunction.

For those men who lose potency, Viagra® (sildenafil), intracavernosal paparavine, and Prostaglandin E1 injections and are very effective. Viagra® has altered the clinical situation considerably. According to one study, for men who are potent at the time of treatment, 92% of patients having seed implants (with or without supplemental external radiation) will maintain erectile function potency. Two additional oral erectile aids, Levitra® (Vardenafil) and Cialis® (Tadalafil) are also now available.

It should also be noted that the risk of erectile dysfunction may be reduced with Palladium-103 because of one of its unique physical properties. The radial dose fall-off, that is, the amount of radiation actually delivered at any distance from the Pd-103 seed, is less with palladium than with any other isotope. Therefore, palladium is less likely to over-radiate the neurovascular bundles or proximal penile tissues, both of which affect the ability to have and maintain an erection.

How do Seed Implants Affect Sexual Activity?

There are no formal restrictions on sexual activity after seed implantation. A patient can resume sexual activities immediately. Some men may not wish to engage in sex right away as the area may be somewhat irritated. As a safety precaution, patients receiving Pd-103 seeds are advised to utilize a condom for a two to three week period after implantation, so as to avoid the unlikely possibility of ejaculating a seed into his partner. That precaution is extended for patients receiving I-125 seeds because of their longer half-life.

For the majority of patients who retain potency, the major change that we see after implantation is the diminution in the volume of the ejaculate. Shortly after the implant, there may also be a discoloring or a different consistency to the ejaculate. Typically it's described as being clearer and thinner, but patients have no problem with that as long as they're able to maintain an erection and achieve orgasm.

A patient can have normal sperm after implantation. The testicles are a separate organ from the prostate per se, and while there may be a short period of oligospermia (a decrease in the sperm count), a patient very well may have a return of sperm. Although there is little chance that radiation will affect the sperm, attempts to impregnate should be avoided for at least 6 months. Because of the diminished ejaculate, and the change in milieu that the sperm will encounter, the chance of successful impregnation is probably greatly reduced, though several of my patients have successfully conceived. We counsel our patients that they need to be careful and should not consider themselves to be sterile because of the procedure. At the same time, men wanting to father children should always consider banking sperm before implantation.

What Precautions Should Patients Exercise after the Implant Procedure?

After implantation, patients are advised for the first month not to hold children less than two years of age for extended periods—for hours in a day or for consecutive days. This applies only to Palladium-103 implants, because that isotope has a short half-life and delivers its dose relatively quickly. With Iodine-125 implants, a longer period of restraint needs to be exercised. These restrictions do not mean having no contact. Even during the period immediately after the implant, a patient can have casual contact with children less than two years old. It's perfectly safe for a seeding patient to hold a child his lap for brief periods.

How are Implants Modified for Patients with Prior TURPs?

If a patient has had a TURP, the implant procedure has to be mapped out very carefully and the seeds need to be distributed differently in that particular patient. They have to be positioned in a way that avoids the TURP itself; otherwise, they may be deposited into an empty prostatic cavity and eventually be urinated out. Misplaced seeds may cause potential damage in that way. With these patients, I use a seed loading pattern that is very peripheral to the gland, placing seeds in extracapsular positions and especially avoid the remaining external sphincter.

The reason that incontinence risks may be high in these patients is because a TURP typically removes the superior internal sphincter, leaving the patient with only the lower sphincter. The high doses of implant radiation may impair that sphincter's ability to work normally. Another factor to consider is how large the TURP is compared to the size of the prostate. There must be enough prostate tissue around the TURP to anchor the seeds; if the TURP is excessive, there may not be enough tissue for the seeds to adhere. That might be a contraindication to seed implantation, though it's rare that a prior TURP would prevent a patient from being seeded.

What are the Advantages of Palladium-103 over Iodine-125?

The choice of palladium versus iodine is typically based on physician preference, although it is sometimes decided by the patient. While there is some controversy regarding which is the superior source, palladium has long been my isotope of choice, a preference dating back to my experience in the mid-1980's with both Pd-103 and I-125 at New York University Medical Center and Memorial Sloan-Kettering. My research and clinical practice in Tampa during the following decade and my more recent experience in Sarasota have confirmed the advantages of Pd-103 in a large brachytherapy practice.

Radiobiological considerations suggest that palladium would be more effective against rapidly growing, more aggressive cancers (those with higher Gleason scores) as well as low-grade prostate malignancies. While there have been no definitive (prospective, randomized) human clinical trials to date comparing tumor-control rates with Pd-103 and I-125, studies have reported a lower complication rate for Pd-103, as well as a more precipitous fall in PSA levels and reduced incidence of benign PSA "bounce" (see below, What is PSA Bounce?).

Why Should Seed Implants be Done
after External Radiation?

When external radiation is combined with brachytherapy, the sequence is typically EBRT (preferably IMRT) followed by an implant boost, with the doses of each modality moderated to achieve optimal coverage while at the same time limiting rectal, bladder and urethral doses. The history of the combined approach suggests there may be considerable reason for concern that reversing the sequence (implant first followed by external radiation) may increase the risk of rectal complications, in part because there is a significant interval when patients are receiving simultaneous implant and external radiation.

We have learned that by targeting the tumor and its extensions first with IMRT, with or without hormonal therapy, the seeding procedure is more effective and serves as a boost, while not leaving the migrating cells in the regions outside of the prostate untreated. The surrounding pelvic field is essentially sterilized and cancers are rendered nonviable when IMRT is used before the seed implantation. Some doctors who have treated in the reverse order, implanting seeds before administering external radiation, have reported higher rates of rectal injury. There is also concern that implanting seeds first in intermediate or high grade cancers may spread cancer into the bloodstream. This potential threat is eliminated with the implant-boost approach, because the external radiation has sterilized the peripheral field prior to the insertion of implant needles.

What is the Likelihood of Cure
with Brachytherapy and IMRT?

The 10-year and 12-year cure rates for brachytherapy or combination therapy using brachytherapy and external radiation (3D-CRT or IMRT) are as good as or better than results achieved with other treatment modalities, including surgical removal of the prostate. Freedom from biochemical failure is typically 90% or higher for low risk patients receiving brachytherapy, while even intermediate and high risk patients may enjoy an approximate 80% freedom from biochemical failure when brachytherapy is combined with external radiation.

The criteria used at my institution for biochemical disease-free survival is quite rigorous. Only patients who achieve and maintain a PSA nadir of 0.2 or less are considered disease-free. After seed implants and external radiation, the prostate is left in place and any remaining normal prostate cells will secrete PSA, so there will be a certain baseline PSA level. I have patients with PSA levels as high as 3.0 that over time have never shown any PSA velocity. Their PSA readings have been stable and not rising for a decade or more; however, when using strict criteria, they are technically not cured, even though most of these patients will probably never have symptoms or die from prostate cancer. As such, the actual cure rate may be somewhat higher than that reported.

What is a PSA Bounce?

About 30% to 40% of patients undergoing seed implantation experience a temporary rise in PSA after an initial decline in their PSA level following treatment. This phenomenon is known as a PSA bounce or flare. It generally occurs approximately 20 months after treatment and is not caused by a recurrence of cancer, but rather by radiation-induced prostatitis (inflammation of the prostate) with subsequent systemic release of PSA. These patients are still considered disease-free. The rise in PSA may be 0.1 or higher and can sometimes last many months, but it is usually of short duration. Studies have shown that the PSA bounce is more common with younger patients, those who receive higher implant doses, and those with larger prostate glands.

How do Brachytherapy and IMRT Compare with Surgery?

As discussed earlier, treatments can be compared in terms of cure rates and complication rates by evaluating the results obtained at premier medical centers for each treatment specialty. For low risk patients, brachytherapy with or without supplemental IMRT (or 3D-CRT) appears to be comparable to surgery as far as likelihood of cure, but with less risk of serious, long-term complications. For intermediate and high risk patients, a number of recent studies have shown brachytherapy and supplemental IMRT (or 3D-CRT) to be significantly more effective at curing prostate cancer than surgery (Figures 12-13).

STATE OF THE ART
BRACHYTHERAPY
AND IMRT

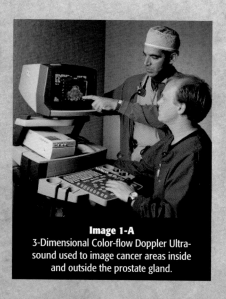

Image 1-A
3-Dimensional Color-flow Doppler Ultrasound used to image cancer areas inside and outside the prostate gland.

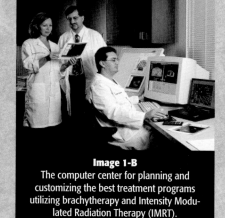

Image 1-B
The computer center for planning and customizing the best treatment programs utilizing brachytherapy and Intensity Modulated Radiation Therapy (IMRT).

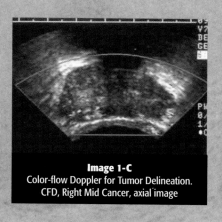

Image 1-C
Color-flow Doppler for Tumor Delineation. CFD, Right Mid Cancer, axial image

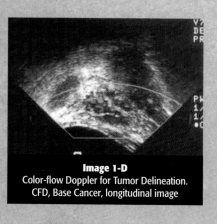

Image 1-D
Color-flow Doppler for Tumor Delineation. CFD, Base Cancer, longitudinal image

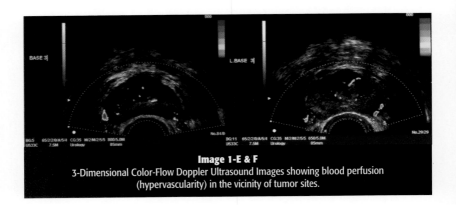

Image 1-E & F
3-Dimensional Color-Flow Doppler Ultrasound Images showing blood perfusion (hypervascularity) in the vicinity of tumor sites.

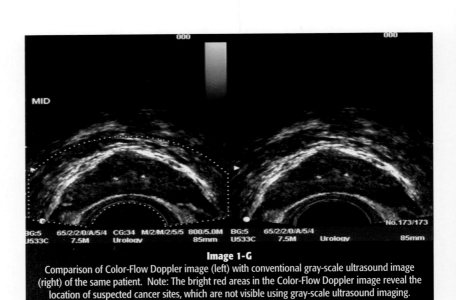

Image 1-G
Comparison of Color-Flow Doppler image (left) with conventional gray-scale ultrasound image (right) of the same patient. Note: The bright red areas in the Color-Flow Doppler image reveal the location of suspected cancer sites, which are not visible using gray-scale ultrasound imaging.

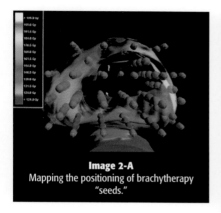

Image 2-A
Mapping the positioning of brachytherapy "seeds."

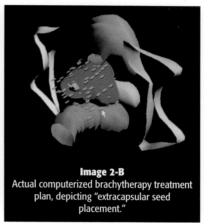

Image 2-B
Actual computerized brachytherapy treatment plan, depicting "extracapsular seed placement."

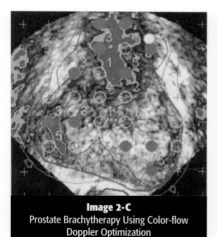

Image 2-C
Prostate Brachytherapy Using Color-flow Doppler Optimization

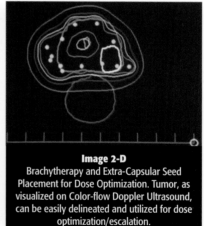

Image 2-D
Brachytherapy and Extra-Capsular Seed Placement for Dose Optimization. Tumor, as visualized on Color-flow Doppler Ultrasound, can be easily delineated and utilized for dose optimization/escalation.

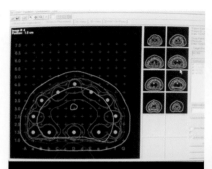

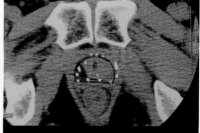

Image 2-E
Brachytherapy Dose Optimization Using Extra-Capsular Seeds. Tumor, as visualized on Color-flow Doppler Ultrasound, can be easily delineated and utilized for dose optimization/ escalation.

Image 2-F
Brachytherapy Dose Optimization. Tumor delineation on post-implant CT for dosimetric analysis.

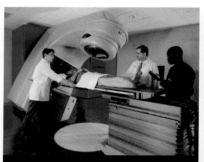

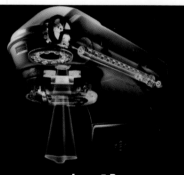

Image 3-A
A modern, digital medical linear accelerator for delivering "Smart Beam" high resolution Intensity Modulated Radiation Therapy (IMRT).

Image 3-B
Inside a medical linear accelerator. The radiation beams pass through and are shaped by a device called a multileaf collimator so that it conforms to the shape of the tumor. Courtesy of Varian Medical Systems.

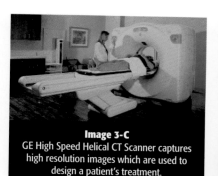

Image 3-C
GE High Speed Helical CT Scanner captures high resolution images which are used to design a patient's treatment.

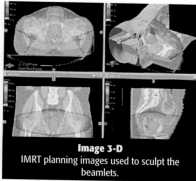

Image 3-D
IMRT planning images used to sculpt the beamlets.

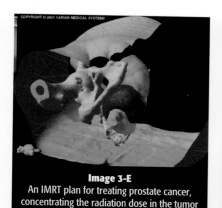

Image 3-E
An IMRT plan for treating prostate cancer, concentrating the radiation dose in the tumor (red) while avoiding the nearby bladder (yellow) and rectum (green). Courtesy of Varian Medical Systems.

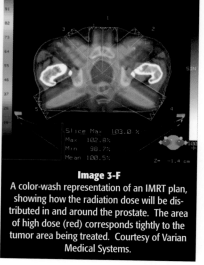

Image 3-F
A color-wash representation of an IMRT plan, showing how the radiation dose will be distributed in and around the prostate. The area of high dose (red) corresponds tightly to the tumor area being treated. Courtesy of Varian Medical Systems.

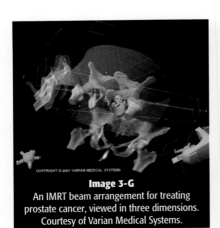

Image 3-G
An IMRT beam arrangement for treating prostate cancer, viewed in three dimensions. Courtesy of Varian Medical Systems.

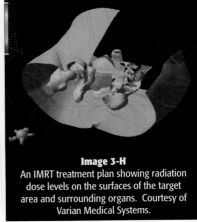

Image 3-H
An IMRT treatment plan showing radiation dose levels on the surfaces of the target area and surrounding organs. Courtesy of Varian Medical Systems.

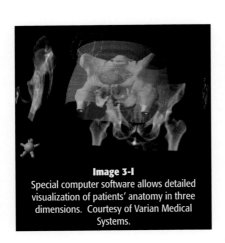

Image 3-I
Special computer software allows detailed visualization of patients' anatomy in three dimensions. Courtesy of Varian Medical Systems.

The results of my own published studies are consistent with those reported by the brachytherapy teams described above, showing a similar plateau in the disease-free curve (Figure 14). My personal series dates from 1991 with Pd-103 seed implantation and supplemental external radiation, utilizing 3D-CRT and more recently IMRT for the treatment of intermediate and high risk patients. The overall actuarial freedom from biochemical failure at 10 years was 79% in patients having locally advanced, high risk prostate cancer. That number is actually improving to more than 80% with

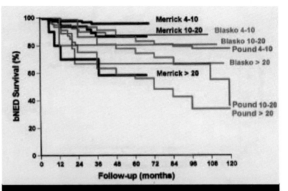

Figure 12–Permanent Prostate Brachytherapy compared to Prostatectomy. Biochemical disease-free (bNED) survival for selected prostatectomy (Chan et al, Pound et al) and brachytherapy series (Blasko et al, Merrick et al) stratified by Gleason score of at least 5 (J of Brachy Int., Vol. 17, July-Sept. 2001, 193).

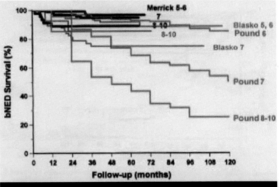

Figure 13–Permanent Prostate Brachytherapy compared to Prostatectomy. Biochemical disease free survival (bNED) for selected prostatectomy (Chan et al, Pound et al) and brachytherapy series (Blasko et al, Merrick et al) stratified by pretreatment prostate specific antigen level (J of Brachy Int., Vol. 17, July-Sept. 2001, 193).

patients who have now been followed for 12 years or more. Meanwhile, morbidity has been limited to temporary urinary symptoms, similar to those that occur with seed implants alone.

A note of caution should be added with regard to seed implants as monotherapy. Back in the 1990's, intermediate risk patients were commonly treated with seeds alone, and now we are seeing a small percentage of these patients experiencing biochemical failure beyond 8 years. This

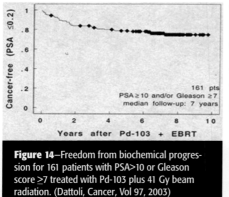

Figure 14—Freedom from biochemical progression for 161 patients with PSA>10 or Gleason score ≥7 treated with Pd-103 plus 41 Gy beam radiation. (Dattoli, Cancer, Vol 97, 2003)

would indicate that the combined approach of seed implants with supplemental external radiation is a more effective protocol for patients at the intermediate risk level.

Our success with higher risk patients is indicative of an important area where brachytherapy and IMRT offer significant advantages over surgery. From a surgical perspective, it's very difficult if not impossible to cure stage T3 malignancies, and it's very difficult to cure patients having Gleason scores in the 7 to 10 range and PSA's greater than 10. But we have had a very successful run using external radiation for about four to five weeks, and then adding the implant boost using Pd-103 brachytherapy about four weeks later. This integrated approach has been able to cure some cancers which were formerly deemed to be incurable with surgery or any other treatment option.

As mentioned, even patients who have evidence of lymph node involvement are now being treated. This group of patients is also treated with hormonal agents. Combined hormone blockade is followed by IMRT to target not only the prostate but also the periprostatic tissues and the lymph node bearing sites. Then finally the seeds are implanted where most of the tumor volume is, namely in the prostate itself. Having treated patients with lymph node cancer successfully, we are moving up the ladder in terms of the stage of the disease that can be conquered.

What are Proton and Neutron Beam Therapies and how do They Compare to Other Forms of Radiation?

Radiation therapy in all its forms utilizes atomic or subatomic particles: electrons, protons, neutrons and photons, which include x-rays and gamma rays. These particles differ in terms of charge, mass and other physical characteristics. Like visible light, the energy of conventional x-ray radiation takes the form of photons. Radiation therapies utilizing proton and neutron beams have been developed in the hope that they might offer some advantage over conventional photon beams. Protons and neutrons are generated by proton accelerators rather than the linear accelerators that are used to generate photons.

Each type of radiation therapy delivers a dose of highly energized particles that interact in various ways with the tissue they traverse. In the case of x-rays and protons, a process called ionization causes electrons to be displaced in the atoms of DNA molecules in cancer cells. This interaction damages the DNA and causes cell death. The strategy of targeting tumors with cancer-killing doses of radiation is essentially the same regardless of which kind of radiation is used.

Unlike other forms of radiation like x-rays that begin releasing their energy as soon as they enter the body, protons travel through bodily tissues initially releasing very little energy, but at a certain calculable point, the energy that the beam delivers rises dramatically to a peak, known as the *Bragg peak*. The Bragg peak is like the focus of a magnifying lens, and allows the radiation to be targeted to the site of the tumor. Protons may have some theoretical advantage over photons because they can be accurately focused to release most of their ionizing energy at a certain depth to encompass a calculated tumor volume, while avoiding nearby healthy organs. By contrast, the depth at which photons deposit their maximal energy is determined by the energy levels of the photons and can range from the skin surface to a depth of approximately 4 centimeters.

The radiobiological effect (RBE) of protons in high doses is nearly identical to the RBE of high-energy photons utilized with IMRT. However, with its highly sophisticated beam arrangements and state-of-the-art prostate immobilization, IMRT allows for the delivery of higher doses than protons. Several published studies have already demonstrated the advantages of IMRT over 3D-CRT at high dose levels, and proton therapy at this time does not deliver higher doses than 3D-CRT. The preponderance of data suggests that higher doses lead to higher cure rates, regardless of the type of radiation utilized. It appears unlikely that researchers using protons will be able to safely escalate doses as high as those now achieved with IMRT, or the even higher doses delivered when IMRT is combined with a seed implant boost.

Proton beam radiation therapy (PBRT) is presently available at only two institutions in the U.S. (Loma Linda Medical Center and Massachusetts General Hospital). PBRT is usually performed on an outpatient basis over a period of 7 to 8 weeks (35 to 40 sessions). Protons are sometimes combined with a reduced course of conventional radiation. Proton therapy is FDA and Medicare approved, and costs are roughly comparable to the more advanced forms of conventional radiation therapy.

Promising 5-year results with PBRT have been reported by physicians at Loma Linda (Slater JD, et al, Int J Radiat Oncol Biol Phys 43: 719-25, 1999). In that study, patients ranged from stage T1 to T3, and as many as 91% of the patients who reached a PSA nadir of less than or equal to 0.5 had no clinical or biochemical evidence of disease. These results are still considered short-term, and the PSA nadir value of 0.5 may be criticized by some researchers as not being strict enough (three rises of 10% or more above that baseline were used to define biochemical failure). Adjusting the figure to a rigorous 0.2 nadir would most likely decrease the success rate to some extent.

Proton therapy causes significantly fewer complications than does traditional external radiation therapy, though its precision in sparing healthy tissues is probably surpassed by IMRT and/or brachytherapy in the most skilled hands. About half of all proton therapy patients experience some urinary discomfort two to three weeks into treatment. Those symptoms usually dissipate two to three weeks after completing therapy. About 20% of patients develop intermittent rectal bleeding, which may occur 9 to 12 months after treatment and persist episodically for a year or two. A proton therapy patient has between a 30% and 50% chance of experiencing problems with potency, roughly equivalent to the results obtained with nerve-sparing prostatectomies. When erectile dysfunction occurs after proton therapy, it usually happens 9 to 12 months after treatment.

The basic effect of ionizing radiation is to disrupt the ability of cells to divide and grow by damaging their DNA strands. With photons and protons, the damage is done primarily by activated radical ions produced by atomic interactions involving electrons orbiting the nucleus of the atom. Because of the nature of these characteristic interactions, photon and proton radiation are referred to as *low linear energy transfer* (low LET) radiation. With neutron radiation, the damage to the DNA is done primarily by nuclear interactions. Neutrons are referred to as *high linear energy transfer* (high LET) radiation. Tumor cells damaged by high LET radiation (neutrons) are less able to repair themselves and continue to grow than are tumor cells damaged by low LET radiation (photons and protons).

In addition, unlike low LET photons and protons, neutrons do not depend on oxygen to damage the DNA in cancer cells and cause cell death. Therefore, neutron beam therapy may have a certain theoretical advantage over conventional photon radiation because high LET neutrons may be more effective against large, bulky tumors that typically have low oxygen levels (hypoxic) near the center of their mass. This characteristic of neutrons might afford some benefit when treating these larger tumors that are more resistant to low LET radiation and to hormonal therapy.

The radiobiological effect of neutrons is so high that the required prescription dose is about one-third the dose required with photons or protons. As such, a full course of neutron therapy is carried out with only 10 to 12 treatments, compared to 30 to 40 treatments needed for conventional x-ray radiation. Neutrons are sometimes combined with a reduced course of standard radiation therapy. 5-year clinical trials of neutrons have suggested that they may be more effective against advanced prostate cancers than is conventional radiation; however, these results are still considered short-term. Because neutrons are such a highly penetrating form of radiation, they may also carry a greater risk of complications than conventional radiation therapy.

Studies with protons and neutrons are not yet definitive and further investigation is warranted with each modality. Both protons and neutrons are now being used as salvage therapies after surgical failure. As the technology continues to evolve, the delivery systems for these alternative forms of radiation are likely to see further refinements that may improve the overall accuracy and effectiveness of each of these therapies.

What are the Treatment Options if External Radiation Fails?

Patients who are not cured by any of the various forms external radiation therapy have several options for salvage therapy, including radical surgery.

As mentioned, the operation to remove the prostate is more difficult after radiation. Many doctors do not recommend salvage prostatectomy because of their own limited experience. They will inform the patient that the risk of complications is high, while the likelihood of cure is relatively low. Nonetheless, this remains a viable option in experienced surgical hands.

A second treatment with radiation is usually not advised since the first course of radiation did not cure the cancer and the risk of complications is high. There has been, however, a growing interest in treating failed external radiation patients with brachytherapy, since seed implant radiation can be focused on the prostate, with less risk of damage to the rectum and surrounding tissue. One recent study reported that as many as 50% of these salvage brachytherapy patients were disease-free at 5 years.

Cryosurgery is a primary treatment method that involves the insertion of freezing probes into the prostate to kill cancerous tissue. This technique has also been used as a salvage therapy for locally recurrent prostate cancer after failed radiation, though there is little published data available. One study reported a disease-free survival rate of 74% after two years, but with a very high rate of complications such as incontinence and erectile dysfunction. This incontinence rate is dramatically reduced in experienced hands (see Chapter Seven).

If a man's PSA after external radiation (or brachytherapy) rises only very slowly over a period of one to three years, then the cancer may still be confined within the prostate. These patients have the most options of patients who fail with radiation, including watchful waiting. A number of studies have shown that there are patients with biopsy-detected local recurrence who have survived 10 years or more without experiencing any progression of the disease. However, more aggressive tumors with Gleason scores of 7 to 10 may secrete little PSA, and even a slow PSA rise may be significant with respect to tumor growth and cancer spread.

In addition to salvage treatments like brachytherapy, surgery and cryosurgery, there are also the options of hormonal therapy or orchiectomy (surgical castration). The same considerations that apply to hormonal therapy after failed surgery apply to hormonal therapy for men with local or distant cancer recurrence after radiation. Some studies suggest that men treated with a combination of hormones and radiation as their initial treatment have a reduced rate of failure. However, initial radical prostatectomy coupled with hormones have not demonstrated a similar benefit.

With the object of shutting down the body's production of testosterone completely, many doctors combine drugs like Lupron® (or Eligard® or Zoladex®) with Casodex® (or Eulexin®), which together provide a total blockage against the male hormones that nourish prostate cancer. For many men, the use of this type of combination hormonal therapy to achieve a castration level of testosterone that may slow the progression of the disease is preferable to undergoing surgical castration (orchiectomy), which is a less expensive way to achieve the same end. In addition, unlike surgical castration, this form of medical castration is reversible and may be used intermittently. The patients may be on hormones 6 to 12 months, and then completely off hormones until the PSA reaches a predetermined value. This allows for recovery of the male bodily functions.

What are the Treatment Options if Brachytherapy Fails?

Patients who have had seed implantation without initial success have the option of being re-seeded. Although long term results are not yet available, this approach appears to be promising, and typically involves using a different isotope the second time around. If the patient was first implanted with iodine, then palladium might be used as a salvage therapy in the hope that the cancer will be more sensitive to the second isotope. If the first implant was technically mishandled, then a second implant affords the opportunity of correcting misplacements that may have caused underdosing. In some cases, HDR temporary implants may be used if permanent implants fail.

Brachytherapy patients who experience treatment failure also have the salvage options of surgery, cryosurgery, hormonal therapy, and watchful waiting. In some cases, several months of hormonal therapy may be prescribed to reduce the size of the tumor prior to an attempt at salvage therapy with either surgery or cryosurgery.

CHAPTER SEVEN

CRYOSURGERY

What is Cryosurgery?

Cryosurgery (also called cryotherapy or cryoablation) uses the process of freezing and thawing to destroy cancer cells. The technique has been in use for some time for the treatment of cervical cancer, as well as malignancies of the head, neck, and skin. Early attempts at prostate cryosurgery were associated with an unacceptably high rate of complications, but the advent of transrectal ultrasound has improved cryosurgical results for the treatment of early stage prostate cancer.

Current cryosurgical technique involves subjecting prostate tissue to extremely cold temperatures (-40° or less) with the use of probes containing liquid nitrogen and more recently Argon gas. The cryoprobes are needles inserted through the perineum and into the prostate gland. The probes create ice balls that destroy both cancerous and normal prostate tissue. The urethra is protected by an indwelling catheter through which a warm saline solution is circulated.

Ultrasound, CT scans or MRI may be used to guide the placement of 6 to 8 probes, and to carefully control the amount of tissue frozen. Temperature probes (thermocouples) within and around the gland monitor the freezing process. The procedure is often repeated two to three times to achieve maximum destruction or ablation of the gland. Several months of hormonal therapy may be used to reduce the size of the gland prior to treatment.

Cryosurgery may offer certain advantages over radical surgery. The freezing procedure does not involve any cutting and is performed on an outpatient basis under local or general anesthesia. Unlike surgery, cryosurgery can be repeated, however, this may not be an advantage, as the object of treatment is to eradicate the cancer initially, once and for all. Many patients are circumspect about a therapy that may only be temporary, and recurrent cancers, when they occur, are typically more aggressive.

Prostate tissue destroyed by the cryosurgery procedure is not removed, but is absorbed by the body. Recovery time is brief, and serious complications in recent years have been comparable to surgery and conventional external beam radiation. Because the procedure typically damages or destroys the neurovascular bundles, most cryosurgery patients are rendered impotent by the procedure. Patients who choose cryosurgery should therefore be prepared to deal with erectile dysfunction.

Another source of concern about cryosurgery stems from the fact that studies have shown that as many as 20% to 30% of patients have cancer that involves the urethra or the tissue immediately surrounding the urethra. Because cryosurgery entails warming the urethra, there is some likelihood that cancer in this area will not be destroyed by the procedure. Additionally, patients who have cancers involving the apex (bottom portion) of the prostate are likely to suffer incontinence since the external sphincter is invariably affected.

What Patients are Eligible for Cryosurgery?

The procedure does not involve much physical stress and is well tolerated by most men, although cryosurgery does typically require two to four hours utilizing techniques such as rectal warming (whereby saline is instilled between the rectum and prostate). Candidates for cryosurgery as a primary treatment should be limited to those patients with early stage prostate cancer (T2 or less). Men with more advanced cancer are less likely to be cured because the cryoprobes are only effective at killing cancer within the prostate and at the periphery of the gland. As discussed previously, cryosurgery is also being used as a salvage therapy for patients with locally recurrent cancer after radiation.

What are the Risks of Complications after Cryosurgery?

As mentioned, most cryosurgery patients experience erectile dysfunction. According to the published reports, the likelihood of other complications varies considerably and probably reflects the skills and experience of the cryosurgeons and differences in the equipment used. The freezing process may damage the bladder and intestines, leading to pain, a burning sensation, and the need to empty the bladder and bowels often. In addition, a fistula (an abnormal opening or passage) between the rectum and bladder develops in about 2% of men after cryosurgery even in experienced hands. This problem may require surgical repair.

Approximately 50% of patients experience swelling of the penis and scrotum after cryosurgery, usually lasting a couple of weeks. Most men recover normal bowel and bladder function. Approximately 10% to 15% of patients experience sloughing of dead tissue into the urethra. When this occurs, a TURP is usually performed to remove the excess tissue in order to prevent urethral blockage. The TURP may increase incontinence rates considerably.

What is the Likelihood of Cure with Cryosurgery?

Early results with cryosurgery have been mixed. There is no long-term data to suggest that cryosurgery is superior to either radiation therapy or surgery. One 5-year multi-institutional study reported no progression of the disease in 45%, 71% and 76% of high, intermediate and low-risk patients respectively—an overall success rate of 63% (Long JP, Bahn D, Lee F, et al, Urology 57:518-523, 2001).

In this study, low risk patients were defined as those with T1 or T2 cancers, PSA less than or equal to 10, and Gleason score less than seven. High risk patients were those having at least two of the following features: a clinical state T2b or greater, PSA higher than 10, Gleason score greater than 6. Intermediate risk patients were defined as those having any one of those three risk features. The authors of the study defined biochemical failure as a post-treatment PSA higher than 1.0. Such a high nadir value suggests that residual cancer may remain in some of those patients who were classified as disease-free. As mentioned, most studies use a post-treatment PSA of 0.5 or less, or even 0.2 or less, to define cure.

It is still too early to judge the true effectiveness of this treatment as a cure for prostate cancer. Some cryosurgeons point out that results have lagged behind refinements in the procedure, such as the recent use of

Argon as a coolant and the use of a template similar to that used for brachytherapy to guide the cryoprobes.   Progress has made evaluation of cryosurgery problematic because the equipment and techniques vary substantially at those centers offering the procedure. Patients who are inclined toward this treatment are advised to choose one of the premier cryosurgeons with published results.

CHAPTER EIGHT

TREATING METASTATIC DISEASE

What Treatments are Used When Cancer Spreads Beyond the Prostate?

When cancer spreads beyond the prostate gland, it generally goes to the pelvic lymph nodes first, and then spreads to distant sites in the body such as the bones. Because of the slow progression of prostate cancer, some men can live for many years even after cancer has metastasized to the lymph nodes or bones. As discussed, significant progress has been made using the combined protocol of brachytherapy and IMRT for treating high risk patients with locally advanced disease (seminal vesicle or regional lymph node involvement).

Unfortunately, once prostate cancer has spread beyond the lymph nodes to the bones or other distant sites, the disease is not considered curable by any of the primary therapies. Patients with metastatic disease are most often treated by hormonal therapy to temporarily halt the progression of the disease and to relieve symptoms. Patients with advanced prostate cancer may also be treated with various investigational drugs and therapies, or they may opt for watchful waiting.

What is Hormonal Therapy and How Does it Work?

Hormonal therapy, or androgen deprivation therapy (ADT), is a standard treatment for those patients whose cancer has spread beyond the prostate gland. At present, nothing works better for advanced prostate cancer than hormonal therapy. If after radiation therapy or surgery or cryosurgery, there is evidence of a rising PSA (biochemical failure) or a positive biopsy, hormonal therapy is likely to be considered.

Increasingly, men with less advanced prostate cancer are also opting for hormonal therapy, either alone or in combination with radiation or surgery. When hormonal intervention is used to downsize the tumor prior to a primary treatment, it is referred to *neoadjuvant* therapy. Some men elect to undergo hormonal therapy instead of a primary therapy (radiation, surgery, or cryosurgery) because of individual health considerations, advanced age, fear of side effects, and so forth.

Hormonal therapy takes a variety of forms, both surgical (orchiectomy) and chemical, which rely on a common strategy for attacking the cancer. It has long been known that prostate cancer is to some extent dependent on and nourished by the male sex hormone, testosterone. This is one of a group of hormones known as androgens. The androgens are responsible for the masculine body changes associated with puberty: growth of body hair, increased muscle mass and genital size, and the deepening of a man's voice. Testosterone also regulates sexual desire, and influences moods and aggressiveness. Like other hormones, testosterone is a chemical released in the body through various biochemical mechanisms and carried in the bloodstream, where it can be detected by a blood test.

Since testosterone stimulates the growth of prostate cancer cells, depleting or ablating the body's testosterone tends to shrink the size of many tumors, specifically, those that are hormone-sensitive. The goal of hormonal therapy is to decrease the production of testosterone in the body, inhibiting the growth and progression of the cancer. These hormone-sensitive prostate cancers essentially are put into remission by the removal of the body's testosterone. In most cases, hormonal therapy will also significantly reduce pain and other symptoms of the disease when it has metastasized. Because hormonal therapy works against the body's production of the male hormones, it might be more accurately described as anti-hormonal therapy.

Erectile dysfunction and loss of sexual desire are likely with almost every form of hormonal therapy. At least 95% of patients lose sexual desire and the ability to have an erection. Some of the newer hormonal agents discussed below have shown some improvement in maintaining sexual function.

While as many as 85% of prostate cancers are responsive to hormonal ablation, individual patient response to hormonal therapy varies widely. For those who initially respond to treatment, control of the disease may last from several months to many years. Two years is the average. As many as 10% of patients with metastatic disease survive for ten years or more, while more than 25% are still alive after five years. 80% of patients experience some relief of pain. However, in most cases, the cancer eventually becomes resistant to treatment, or *refractory,* and the patient will experience a relapse of the disease. This occurs because some of the cancer cells mutate and become *androgen-independent,* meaning that they are unaffected by male hormones. At this point, no form of hormonal therapy is likely to have a significant impact on the disease. Patients with androgen-independent prostate cancer (AIPC) can still resort to other forms of treatment, including chemotherapy and various chemical agents, which are often administered through clinical trials (see "What options are available once hormonal therapy stops working?").

In our practice we utilize a variety of regimes which may slow or stop prostate cancer growth, with chemotherapy considered as a last resort. These regimes for patients with advanced disease may include agents such as Casodex®, Dostinex®, Avodart®, estrogenic agents, Thalidomide, as well as bone integrity protocols, Cox-II inhibiters, agents which disrupt the IGF-1 pathway disruption, and Ketoconozole. Some of these are discussed in greater detail below.

How Does Hormonal Therapy Kill Cancer Cells?

Androgen deprivation causes what is known as programmed cell death, or *apoptosis,* which affects those cancer cells that are hormone-dependent. This results from a biochemical process referred to as *enzymatic DNA degradation.* Enzymes (often called "suicide enzymes") in the cell break down the genetic memory code and cause the cell to die. The mechanism of programmed cell death involves a long, complicated chain of biochemical events within each cell. Exactly how this process takes place is under continuing study by researchers who are seeking to develop more effective chemical agents to treat the disease. The challenge is to develop agents that kill the cancer cells without harming healthy prostate cells.

What is an Orchiectomy?

A bilateral orchiectomy involves the surgical removal of the testicles from the scrotum. This procedure is also known as surgical castration. While the idea of castration makes most men uncomfortable, orchiectomy is the quickest, surest way to reduce the level of testosterone. It is a palliative rather than curative treatment, aimed at easing symptoms rather than curing the underlying cause of the symptoms. Orchiectomy is one of several hormonal options for patients with late stage prostate cancer, though for most patients, it is the least appealing.

The testicles produce about 95 percent of the body's testosterone, and after their removal, a dramatic impact is often observed on the cancer, with a marked fall in the serum PSA level. Orchiectomy usually results in a retardation of the growth and spread of the cancer. Most tumors (both primary and metastases) shrink in size after a bilateral orchiectomy is performed. Patients also experience a significant alleviation of pain and other symptoms. In most cases, the benefits of orchiectomy will be temporary, and eventually the disease will reassert itself. Nevertheless, the procedure may stave off the symptomatic effects of the disease for many months or years.

The operation is minor and can be performed on an out-patient basis, using general or local anesthesia. However, many men find this surgery difficult to accept, even those patients who are no longer sexually active. The side effects associated with castrate testosterone levels vary considerably from patient to patient. Although most men will experience loss of sexual desire and impotence following a bilateral orchiectomy, as many as 10% of patients retain sexual function. Hot flashes are a common side effect of the operation, affecting about one third of patients. Hot flashes involve a sudden rush of heat to the face, neck, upper chest, and back, lasting from a few seconds to an hour. These symptoms can be counteracted or ameliorated by various medications.

Orchiectomy may also cause mood changes, such as irritability or a loss of aggressiveness. Loss of muscle mass, weight gain, bone loss (osteopenia and osteoporosis) and changes in skin tone and hair growth are frequently reported as late effects of treatment. Compared to other forms of hormonal therapy, a major disadvantage of bilateral orchiectomy is that it is irreversible. A small minority of men will have a form of prostate cancer that is hormonally independent, and do not respond to the procedure. These men derive no benefit from the operation. Less than 20% of patients choose orchiectomy over other forms of hormonal therapy.

What is Estrogen Therapy?

The administration of the female hormone, estrogen, inhibits the production of testosterone. Until recent years, this was the most common form of androgen deprivation therapy. When the pituitary gland in the brain detects the presence of female hormones, it stops production of male hormones by the testicles. Estrogenic compounds block the signal transmitted by the pituitary gland, known as luteinizing hormone (LH), which normally stimulates testosterone production. In the past, the most commonly prescribed form of estrogen was diethylstilbestrol, or DES®, taken orally. DES® is cheaper than most other hormone medications, but is no longer commonly prescribed because of the risk of blood clots. However, this risk is effectively countered by using blood thinners such as Coumadin. Estrogens have for the most part been replaced by LHRH agonists and anti-androgens, although estrogens remain an option when LHRH agonists and anti-androgens cease to work (see "What is LHRH therapy?").

Studies have shown DES® to be as effective as orchiectomy for temporarily halting the progression of prostate cancer. However, like orchiectomy, there are a number of side effects associated with estrogen therapy. These include fluid retention, breast enlargement and tenderness (gynecomastia), loss of sexual desire and erectile dysfunction, and rarely nausea and vomiting. Even more serious, estrogen therapy may result in severe circulatory or thrombotic problems, such as blood clots and stroke.

Aside from DES®, other drugs that have been used for estrogen therapy include Premarin® and ethinyl estradiol, which are medications also used by some women during menopause. In my practice, transdermal patches such as Estraderm® and Climara® are used to avoid metabolism of estrogen within the liver, and thereby reduce the risk of dangerous thrombotic side effects. For some men with advanced cancer who do not respond to other estrogen drugs, symptomatic relief may be achieved with polyestradiol phosphate (Stilphostrol®), which is given intravenously. Polyestradiol intramuscular (Estradurin®) may also be prescribed, administered by monthly injection. Another estrogen drug sometimes prescribed is estramustine phosphate (EMCYT®), which is taken orally, but it too carries the risk of serious side effects. PC SPES™ is an herbal form of hormonal therapy that was used until recently when the product was found to contain DES® and/or Coumadin and/or Indomethacin.

What is LHRH Therapy?

This form of hormonal therapy utilizes *leutinizing hormone releasing hormone* (LHRH) agonists (or analogs), a synthesized form of a natural brain hormone. LHRH agonists effectively shut down production of testicular testosterone, achieving the same effect as surgical removal of the testicles. LHRH agonists currently available in the U.S. include leuprolide (Lupron®, Viadur®, and Eligard®), goserelin (Zoladex®), and triptorelin (Trelstar LA®). LHRH agonists may be injected monthly or every 3, 4, or 12 months in the physician's office.

LHRH therapy has been a great benefit to those men who wish to avoid surgery and the deleterious side effects of estrogen therapy. However, LHRH therapy is not without its disadvantages. The drugs are expensive, as they can cost $350 or more per month, which may be prohibitively high for some patients, although most insurance companies cover the cost in full. The side effects of LHRH agonists are similar to those associated with bilateral orchiectomy, namely hot flashes, some loss of libido, weight-gain, and in some cases erectile dysfuncton. Infrequent gastrointestinal side effects have been reported as well.

A "flare reaction" is observed when LHRH therapy is initiated, causing a brief rise or surge in testosterone level. The testosterone flare is accompanied by a rise in PSA and subsequent exacerbation of cancer symptoms, such as bone pain and urinary difficulties in some men. This initial phase typically lasts only a week or two. Small doses of estrogenic compounds, or *anti-androgens* such as flutamide (Eulexin®), bicalutamide (Casodex®), nilutamide (Nilandron®), and cyproterone acetate (Androcur®) may be administered 7 days prior to the initiation of LHRH therapy, as they act to block this flare phenomenon. The anti-androgens prevent attachment of testosterone to prostate cells, and they are used to block the small percentage of testosterone produced by the adrenal glands.

The anti-androgen drugs may also cause side effects such as breast enlargement and nipple tenderness. These problems can be avoided by a short course of radiation therapy administered to the breast tissue. About 10% of men experience nausea and/or diarrhea when taking anti-androgens. There is also some small risk of liver damage, and therefore, a blood test to check liver enzymes is usually given every three months.

A newer hormonal agent, abarelix (Plenaxis®), is known as a a gonadotropin-releasing hormone (GnRH) antagonist. Abarelix has been show to induce castration-level testosterone without the temporary testosterone surge associated with drugs like Lupron®, Zolodex®, Trelstar LA®, and Viadur®. Often prescribed for patients with bone metastases, Abarelix also reduces pain and urinary symptoms. However, a small percentage of men (less than 5%) have serious allergic reactions to the drug. Abarelix is administered by injection every 2 weeks for the first month, and every 4 weeks thereafter. Patients are monitored for a half hour after being injected to be sure they do not show signs of allergic reaction.

What is Combined Hormonal Therapy?

This form of treatment combines the use of LHRH agonists (or orchiectomy) with an anti-androgen, or with both an anti-androgen and *5-alpha reductase inhibitor,* usually finasteride (Proscar®) or dutasteride (Avodart®). In the prostate gland, 5-alpha reductase is an enzyme that converts testosterone into a more potent growth stimulator or metabolite, dihydrotestosterone (DHT). This enzyme is blocked by the 5-alpha reductase inhibitors such as Proscar®, thus inhibiting the production of DHT. Many researchers now believe that the 5-alpha reductase inhibitors improve the efficacy of hormonal therapy.

A recent National Cancer Institute study has demonstrated that Proscar® actually prevents cancer for 25% of those patients taking the drug. That same study also reported that Proscar® encouraged more aggressive cancers in a small percentage of men, but that finding has since been refuted. It appears that tissue biopsies of those receiving Proscar® were falsely interpreted as being more aggressive.

Other recent studies have indicated that combination hormonal blockade is superior to other forms of hormonal therapy, extending the average period of remission by several months. In addition, the percentage of patients who respond to therapy is higher, and more men experience complete remission. However, clinical evaluation has been somewhat contradictory concerning the advantages of combination therapy over monotherapy (the use of a single hormonal regimen to suppress androgen production).

A modified combination therapy that uses flutamide (Eulexin®) with finasteride (Proscar®) allows many men to preserve potency while undergoing hormonal therapy. This limited combination of hormones (often referred to as Sequential Androgen Blockade, or SAB) can preserve quality of life, as neither of these drugs impact on sexual function to the extent that other hormonal agents do.

The mechanism of the SAB combination acts to block testosterone (and its more potent metabolite, DHT) on the cellular level of the tumor, while maintaining normal testosterone levels in the bloodstream, with the hope that the patient's sexual function will be preserved. However, with this approach there is a risk of breast enlargement and hypersensitivity of the nipples. These side effects can be counteracted by a short course radiation delivered to the breast before starting therapy, or by administering drugs such as tamoxifen (Nolvadex®) or anastrozole (Arimidex®) to relieve the symptoms after they appear. A variation of this sequential approach substitutes bicalutamide (Casodex®) for flutamide to achieve the same end. Another approach using Casodex® at three times the typical daily dose (150 mg daily) achieves similar results without the dramatic impact on bone integrity and sexual dysfunction.

What is Intermittent Hormonal Therapy?
Intermittent hormonal therapy is a technique currently under investigation that offers the advantage of sparing patients side effects during intervals when they go off therapy. As previously noted, nearly all prostate cancers treated with androgen deprivation therapy become resistant to this treatment over a period of months or years. Some researchers believe that constant androgen suppression may not be necessary, so they recommend intermittent (on-again, off-again) therapy.

With this approach, combination hormonal therapy (an LHRH agonist and an anti-androgen, plus or minus Proscar® or Avodart®) may be utilized for at least six months or more, and then stopped once the patient's PSA drops to an undetectable level. If the PSA level begins to rise to a predetermined value (e.g. 5 to 10), the drugs are started again. The off-phase of therapy can range from several months to several years or more, during which time patients can recover potency and quality of life. The resumption of the body's production of testosterone eventually restores normal blood testosterone levels and resolves most side effects caused by hormonal therapy; however, recovery time varies, and some patients are slow to recover their natural testosterone production.

How are Patients Monitored with Hormonal Therapy?

Patients are typically monitored every six months with a digital rectal exam, a PSA test, and chemistries to test for kidney function and liver function. If the PSA begins to rise, patients are given a bone scan once or twice a year to test for bone metastases. A blood test will also be used to measure the level of testosterone, to be sure it is within the castrate range and not fluctuating. With anti-androgens (Casodex®, flutamide), a blood test for liver enzymes is usually performed every 6 to 8 weeks. In addition, a number of medications are commonly prescribed to ensure bone integrity, in which case, calcium and magnesium levels require monitoring.

What Determines How Long Hormonal Therapy is Effective?

The benefits of hormonal therapy vary considerably from patient to patient. 10% of patients with advanced metastatic disease live longer than ten years. On the other hand, 10% live less than 6 months. Most patients fall somewhere in between, with 50% surviving three years or less.

Two factors appear to determine how long hormonal therapy is effective: the number of hormone-sensitive cells compared to the number of hormone-independent cells, and how fast the cancer is growing (the rate at which the cancer doubles in size). It is the hormone-independent cells that are ultimately fatal, and therefore, the rate at which they are growing is crucial. Research in the field is now focused on controlling these hormone-resistant cancer cells. If you are just beginning hormonal therapy today, it is entirely possible that new treatments will be available by the time hormones have ceased to work for you.

When Should Hormonal Therapy be Initiated?

During recent years there has been a growing enthusiasm for the early initiation of hormonal therapy, especially combination hormonal therapy. Early initiation means starting hormonal therapy before any symptoms of metastatic disease appear. Advocates of this approach point to those studies that indicate some degree of local control achieved with hormonal agents, slowing progression of the disease. It might appear to be common sense that because hormonal therapy lowers PSA, shrinks tumors and slows progression of the cancer, that it would also prolong life. But this may not be the case. Although the benefits of hormonal therapy for treating prostate cancer have been established, there is considerable controversy about how effective hormonal therapy may be at increasing survival.

Researchers remain divided on the optimal time to begin therapy, though recent studies favor early versus late initiation of hormonal therapy. The argument against early use of hormones rests on the fact that those who opt for early initiation will not be able to use hormonal therapy later when symptoms appear. By that time, the tumor may have become androgen-independent and refractory. After the beneficial effects of hormonal therapy have run their course, a patient's cancer may begin to grow again and eventually progress to what it would have been had hormonal therapy never been given. With this in mind, some doctors encourage men with advanced disease to embark on a course of watchful waiting, arguing that these patients should avoid side effects as long as possible since the treatment has not been shown to substantially prolong life. This conservative strategy calls for the use of hormone therapy only if and when symptoms appear.

Other researchers argue that men with smaller tumors and low Gleason scores (less aggressive cancer) might be cured if treatment is started sooner because these patients have less cancer to begin with and slower growing cancer. As a tumor grows and becomes bulky, genetic changes may take place within the cancer cells that lead to androgen-independence; therefore, early treatment might offer some advantage for these patients by attacking the cancer before it becomes refractory. This point of view appears to be supported by a Mayo Clinic non-randomized study which indicated that patients with positive lymph nodes and low Gleason scores lived longer if they were treated hormonally before symptoms appeared.

Early stage patients should also be aware that the survival benefits of hormonal therapy have not been established. Early initiation of hormonal therapy may indeed halt disease progression temporarily while these patients evaluate other primary treatment options. But a number of studies have demonstrated that early hormonal intervention prior to radical surgery does not reduce the risk of biochemical failure. However, the early use of hormones appears to be more advantageous before undertaking radiation as a primary therapy. My own data does not demonstrate a strong advantage to utilizing hormones prior to radiation in patients having high risk features. Nonetheless, my patients who received hormones had far more aggressive tumors, and yet they fared similarly to those low risk patients who did not receive hormones. As the high risk group would have been expected to fare much worse, this would therefore support the use of hormones in this group. In addition, numerous multi-institutional studies both in the U.S. and abroad have demonstrated a benefit with the utilization of hormonal therapy prior to radiation.

It is clear that more men regardless of the stage of their cancer are choosing to initiate hormonal therapy early because of a perceived possibility of cure, or long-term remission. This option may seem appealing given the steady progress in the field and the likely development of new and more effective chemical agents in the near future. However, before making this choice, patients should fully investigate the potential side effects and changes in quality of life that can be anticipated with hormonal manipulation. Men who opt for early combination hormonal therapy should also keep in mind that the hormones are likely to stop working eventually.

Hormonal therapy continues to be controversial because there are still so many unanswered questions in this area, and because doctors disagree about what the answers will turn out to be. The nature of this controversy makes it all the more important for patients to question their doctors carefully before embarking on treatment. Be sure your doctor has considerable experience with hormonal therapy, and find out what that experience has been with other patients of similar age and stage of cancer as your own. You should carefully discuss the pros and cons of each drug with your doctors and if you remain in doubt, by all means, obtain a second opinion. While the lack of definitive knowledge about hormonal therapy may be unsettling, each patient can still make an educated decision based on the possible benefits and risks associated with this form of treatment.

What Options are Available Once Hormonal Therapy Stops Working?

All combinations of hormonal therapy should be completely exhausted before further options are considered. For example, if the anti-androgen Eulexin® ceases to be effective, as indicated by a rising PSA, consideration might be given to changing to Casodex®, or another anti-androgen such as Nilandron® or Androcur®. After patients with advanced disease have exhausted all of these hormonal measures, alternative options may include chemotherapy and clinical trials that offer experimental treatments such as immunotherapy and vaccine therapies.

What are the Pros and Cons of the Various Hormonal Therapies?

Orchiectomy

Pros
1. Easy, quick, effective surgery
2. No ongoing drug therapy
3. Relatively inexpensive ($2000–$3500) compared to drugs

Cons
1. Psychological impact of castration
2. Does not supress adrenal androgens
3. Side effects of impotence, loss of libido, hot flashes
4. Irreversible procedure
5. Loss of bone integrity

Estrogen

Agents include DES®, Estraderm®, Climara®, Stilphostrol®, Estra-durin®, and PS SPES™.

Pros

1. As effective as orchiectomy at achieving castrate-level testosterone
2. Relatively inexpensive compared to other hormonal drugs
3. Requires no surgery

Cons

1. Risk of cardiovascular problems (heart attack, stroke, blood clots)
2. Loss of sexual libido, hot flashes, fluid retention
3. Breast enlargement and/or tenderness
4. Does not supress adrenal androgens

LHRH Agonists

Agents include Lupron®, Zoladex®, Trelstar LA®, and Viadur®.

Pros

1. As effective as orchiectomy, without surgery
2. Low risk of cardiovascular problems
3. Fewer menopausal side effcts than estrogen

Cons

1. Expensive ($4000 to $6000 annually)
2. Risk of tumor flare
3. High risk of erectile dysfunction and loss of libido
4. Hot flashes
5. Skin rash and irritation at injection site
6. Does not suppress adrenal androgens
7. Loss of bone integrity

Anti-androgens

Agents include Eulexin®, Casadex®, Nilandron®, and Androcur®.

Pros

1. Block adrenal androgens
2. Do not require surgery
3. Lower risk of testosterone flare caused by LHRH analogs
4. May increase survival in combination with orchiectomy, or LHRH analogs, or estrogen

Cons

1. Expensive ($4000 to $5000 annually)
2. Diarrhea (10%, especially with flutamide)
3. Small risk of liver toxicity (requiring monitor)
4. Some risk of breast enlargement and/or tenderness

What is Chemotherapy and How Effective is it in Treating Prostate Cancer?

Chemotherapy involves the use of potent toxins (*cytotoxic* agents) to treat cancer. These chemical substances are typically poisonous to both malignant and benign cells. Certain types of cancer such as leukemias and lymphomas are sensitive to relatively low doses of chemotherapy and can be cured by such drugs. Unfortunately, with the drugs that are currently available, chemotherapy is not usually effective in treating prostate cancer. Generally, about 25% of patients with metastatic prostate cancer respond to chemotherapy temporarily, though some of the more recent chemotherapy agents have shown somewhat better results. After administering the drugs, the tumors may shrink to some degree, but the shrinkage usually lasts only a few months, at which point the disease continues to progress.

The choice of whether or not to initiate chemotherapy is one that is made on a case by case basis by each patient in partnership with his doctor. Chemotherapy is typically limited to patients who do not respond or have become resistant to hormonal therapy. Since there is some chance that chemotherapy can bring about temporary remission of the cancer, many patients with advanced disease consider enrolling in clinical trials. These experimental studies provide data that will enable researchers to make better use of chemical agents in the future (See "How are clinical trials conducted and which patients are eligible?").

Some progress is being made by combining chemotherapy agents with other therapies to increase the likelihood that the cancer will shrink and to prolong the amount of time disease progression is interrupted. One recent study has reported promising 10-year results combining chemical agents (vinblastine, doxorubicin, and mitomycin) with radiation and hormonal therapy for the treatment of stage T3 (extracapsular extension) and N1 cancers (lymph node involvement). This study concludes, "The addition of chemotherapy to hormonal and radiation therapy is feasible and is accepted by most men when they are openly informed of their prognosis with conventional therapy" (Bagley CM et al: *Cancer. 2002 May 15; 94(10):2728-32)*. It should be noted that the patients in this study did not have distant metastases. It is not clear whether the results (greater than 70% biochemical disease-free progression) are superior to those achieved with hormonal therapy plus radiation alone, but as the authors point out, larger randomized studies are warranted.

What Chemical Agents are Currently Under Investigation?

Cytotoxic agents are the standard treatment for prostate cancer that does not respond to hormonal manipulation. There are numerous drugs in this class, and their side effects vary considerably. Attempts are being made to more effectively target cytotoxic agents to tumor sites, allowing for increased drug levels and cell death in cancerous tissues while minimizing toxicity for healthy tissues.

The following chemical agents and experimental therapies are among those being used for the treatment of advanced prostate cancer:

CYTADREN® (aminoglutethimide), usually administered in combination with hydrocortisone, selectively inhibits adrenal production of male hormones. Response rates in patients who have failed initial hormonal therapy are generally poor, although some patients have responded favorably to this therapy, with PSA levels falling 50% or more over periods of 2 to 6 months.

HYDROCORTISONE and other steroids fall into the category of endocrine therapies that work to decrease the receptivity of the cell's androgen receptor, thereby decreasing adrenal androgens. Steroids can cause excessive bone loss and usually require the use of bone supplements.

NIZORAL® (ketoconazole) is an antifungal agent that acts to inhibit male hormone production. Some positive results temporarily reducing PSA levels have been achieved using Nizoral® in patients whose cancers have become resistant to standard hormonal therapy.

VELBAN (vinblastine) is a chemotherapy drug being studied in combination with other agents such as the estrogenic compound, estramustine phosphate (Emcyt®), for treating hormone-refractory prostate cancer. Clinical trials with this combination have reported temporary PSA decreases of 50% or more in a significant number of patients.

PROGESTINS such as hydroxyprogesterone caproate, megestrol acetate, and medrogestone, inhibit testosterone production, and have resulted in limited, temporary responses in some patients. These drugs are being studied in combination with other chemotherapy agents in a number of ongoing clinical trials.

TAXANES such as Taxotere® (docetaxel) and Taxol® (paclitaxel) are a class of drugs that have been used in treating breast and ovarian cancers as well as prostate cancer since the 1990's. These and similar drugs are showing increasing efficacy in temporarily improving quality of life for patients with metastatic disease. Many researchers believe this type of chemotherapy will give way to or complement more promising immunologic and angiogenesis therapies (see below).

SURAMIN is a growth factor inhibiting agent under investigation for the treatment of hormone-refractory prostate cancer. Early results were promising, with response rates as high as 70%, but subsequent randomized tests have been less impressive with only about 20% of patients showing reduced PSA levels over a period of months and a reduction in pain associated with bone metastases. The National Cancer Institute is currently sponsoring clinical trials combining suramin with Cytadren®.

APTOSYN® (exisulind) is a drug that has shown some promise in clinical trials and is undergoing further testing. It acts by directing cancerous tissue to undergo programmed cell death (apoptosis) without damaging healthy tissue. One study at Columbia University evaluated the effects of Aptosyn® on locally recurrent prostatectomy patients and found the drug slowed PSA doubling time, suggesting that the initiation of hormonal therapy might be delayed for these patients. Other trials are now underway combining Aptosyn® with Taxotere® for the treatment of hormone-refractory prostate cancer.

PROVENGE® is an immunologic or "vaccine" therapy that directs the body's immune system to destroy cancer cells. Trials are currently underway to test a number of immunologic therapies on patients with hormone-refractory prostate cancer. This approach takes advantage of the fact that the body has cells that are programmed to destroy foreign targets (antigens). Vaccine therapies treat cancer as if it were a foreign agent invading the body, something analogous to a bacterial infection. The goal of researchers is to stimulate the patient's immune system with antigens that mimic the antigens of the cancer cell, thereby causing the immune system to attack the cancer.

ATRASENTAN® is an agent known as an ET *receptor antagonist,* which acts to block a prostate cancer cell product (Endothelin-1 or ET-1) that stimulates *osteoblastic metastases* (bone lesions). ET-1 also acts to constrict blood vessels (vasoconstriction) that may account for bone pain in patients with metastatic cancer. Early results with Atrasentan have shown some promise in slowing disease progression, especially in patients with skeletal metastases. Clinical trials are ongoing and further information can be obtained from Abbott Laboratories in Illinois by contacting their Web site: http://abbott.com/innovation/innovation center.html

COX-II INHIBITORS are a class of drugs that include Celebrex®, widely used as an arthritis medication. The Cox-II inhibitors have shown promise in clinical trials for treating a number of genitourinary cancers, including prostate cancer. Cox-II inhibitors relieve pain, inflammation, and swelling by blocking the body's production of an enzyme called Cox-II. A number of studies are underway to evaluate the effectiveness of these drugs in slowing or preventing the progression of prostate cancer.

ANGIOSTATIN and ENDOSTATIN are agents that act on the molecular level to inhibit the growth of blood vessels that allow tumors to grow and metastasize. In order for tumors to grow, they require nutrients supplied through a network of capillaries. The process by which tumors establish this network of blood vessels is known as *angiogenesis*. Agents like angiostatin and endostatin that interfere with angiogenesis are being tested both as single agents and in combination with other therapies in the hope that such strategies can destroy both androgen-dependent and androgen-independent tumors.

THALIDOMIDE is another agent that acts as an angiogenesis inhibitor, and it may also inhibit COX-II induction. There has been a resurgence of interest in Thalidomide since the 1960's when it was found to cause birth defects. A number of clinical trials have shown promising results in treating androgen-independent prostate cancer. One study of Thalidomide administered as sole agent showed a PSA decline of 50% or more in 18% of patients, and a PSA decline of 40% or more in 27% of patients (Figg W.D. et al, *Clinical Cancer Research, July 2001, Vol. 7, 1888-1893)*. Thalidomide is also being studied in combination with various cytotoxic chemotherapy agents.

ONCOLYTIC VIRUSES are man-made anti-cancer agents produced through genetic engineering. Viruses can be used to transfer genes into a cancer cell. Genetic manipulation allows these viruses to selectively destroy cancer cells by inducing cell death, or *lysis*. There are a number of specific oncolytic viruses under investigation, with names like Cell Genesys Viruses CG7060 and CG7870, Reolysin®, and ONYX-15.

Another strategy utilizing viruses has been to engineer viral strains that can actually restore cancer cells to normal by infusing corrective genetic information, replacing defective genes and thereby rectifying the uncontrolled cell growth that is characteristic of malignant cells. Gene therapy also targets specific genes or proteins such as bcl-2 or p-53, which are involved with the process of programmed cell death.

ANTISENSE THERAPY is a type of gene therapy that involves the use of synthetic DNA and RNA segments called *oligonucleotides* to stop or interrupt the production of cancer-related proteins. Antisense compounds block the transmission of genetic information between the nucleus and protein production sites within the cell, inhibiting genes that are responsible for cancer growth and for resistance to drug therapies. Antisense olignonucleotides targeting the bcl-2 protein has been shown to induce apoptosis and enhance chemosensitivity when used in combination with agents like paclitaxel (Taxol®).

New anti-cancer agents are continuously under development. Several are not mentioned here because research findings into the efficacy of the agents have yet to be made public. With our increasing knowledge regarding the molecular and cellular mechanisms by which prostate cancer progresses, it is very likely that new agents with improved therapeutic potential will be available in the near future.

How are Clinical Trials Conducted and Which Patients are Eligible?

When traditional avenues of treatment are exhausted, men with advanced disease may wish to consider participating in a clinical trial. Trials generally test new treatments and compare them with traditional therapies. They are usually not undertaken as a primary treatment, but may be appropriate for patients with limited therapeutic options. The purpose of a trial is to benefit the patient, whether by prolonging life, improving quality of life, or alleviating pain. If you are considering enrolling in a clinical trial, you should carefully investigate the proposed treatment to be sure you meet the eligibility requirements, as eligibility varies from program to program.

Clinical trials are carried out in three phases. Phase I trials are used to determine doses and toxicity of new drugs and therapies. After the optimal dose is determined, a Phase II trial will be carried out with a limited number of patients to evaluate the effectiveness of the drug or therapy. Before a new drug or therapy becomes FDA-approved, a Phase III trial will be conducted to compare the effectiveness of the newly developed treatment to currently available treatments within a larger population.

If you decide to pursue a clinical trial, you will want to find out whether you are going to receive the new drug or therapy, or instead be part of a double-blind study in which a control or placebo group does not receive the new medication or therapy. If patients fail to receive a benefit from a drug because they are part of a placebo group, they are usually given the drug at the end of the trial. Patients are advised not to give up the opportunity for an established treatment of known effectiveness in favor of a clinical trial in which the efficacy of the new therapy is unknown.

Clinical trials are often conducted by comprehensive medical centers, which develop and test new therapies and therapeutic agents. Trials are also organized by pharmaceutical companies in response to an FDA request to establish the value and safety of a particular drug before it can be marketed. Patients may wish to contact one or more of the comprehensive medical centers located in their area. In the Northeast, some of the premier medical centers include Memorial Sloan-Kettering, Johns Hopkins, Dana Farber, and Columbia. Baylor University and M.D. Anderson are in the south, and the University of Michigan is in the Midwest. West coast centers include UCLA and the University of California in San Francisco. For further information on clinical trials, patients are encouraged to contact the National Cancer Institute's Cancer Information Service at 1-800-4-CANCER, or their Web site: http://cis.nci.nih.gov/

What Therapies Can Alleviate Pain for Patients with Advanced Cancer?

Patients should never hesitate to discuss pain and other quality of life concerns with their doctors. There are a number of effective therapies for relieving pain and most other symptoms associated with prostate cancer and the side effects of treatment. Alleviating pain will allow you not only to concentrate and to make decisions about your treatment, but will also enable you to continue to enjoy life and the things that matter most to you.

When properly prescribed, pain medications including narcotic drugs (opioids) can be very effective. External radiation therapy is utilized as a palliative therapy to relieve pain in patients with metastatic disease. Other forms of radiation are also used to alleviate pain. Samarium-153 (Quadramet®) and Strontium-89 Chloride (Metastron®) are FDA-approved radiopharmaceuticals administered by injection. They go directly to the sites of metastatic bone disease to relieve pain symptoms. A single injection of either of these radioisotopes may alleviate pain for three to six months, after which, the patient can receive repeat injections at intervals of 90 days or more when medically appropriate.

Bisphosphonate compounds, such as Actonel®, Fosamax®, Actonel®, and Aredia®, are drugs that can relieve pain caused by cancer that has metastasized to the bones and may also retard the growth of these metastases. Zoledronic acid (Zometa®) was the first bisphosphonate approved for use in bone metastases caused by prostate cancer. Other bisphosphonates have been approved for other medical uses, and some doctors prescribe them "off label" (a drug prescribed to treat a condition for which it has not been FDA approved) to treat prostate cancer. These substances have an anti-cancer effect and also help prevent or correct bone loss (osteopenia and osteoporosis), which is an unwanted complication of hormonal therapy.

PART TWO

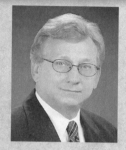

BY DON KALTENBACH

Before deciding on treatment, you may benefit from talking to other patients. The fact is that most patients see things, feel things, and experience things differently than doctors do. Because medical training emphasizes the treatment of disease, doctors sometimes forget they are treating patients, and not just a disease. By joining a support group in your area, you can talk to patients who have been through surgery, radiation, cryosurgery, and hormonal therapy. Listen to what they have to say about

THE PATIENT'S POINT OF VIEW

their experiences, but keep in mind that your situation may be different from theirs.

As you gather information, you will need to use your own best judgment based on the specifics of your case and your own personal needs. Much of the challenge in deciding on the best course of treatment is to become informed about your options, but there are also a number of important emotional and financial considerations that should not be neglected. My own personal history is offered here only as one case in point, with the hope that the lessons I have learned over the years may help you come to grips with some of the immediate and long-term challenges you may face.

CHAPTER NINE

ONE PATIENT'S JOURNEY

The Shock of Discovery

The year was 1990, and I was 44 years old, in my prime and much younger than most men are when diagnosed with prostate cancer. During the previous year, I had gone through some dramatic changes in my life, all of them very positive. After working for almost two decades as a lawyer in the town of New Port Richey, Florida, my practice was flourishing and I was building a new office. At the same time, my wife Nancy and I had a new baby on the way, which seemed almost miraculous given the circumstances that led to her pregnancy.

Nancy and I had been trying for years to have a baby, but without success. Eventually, we both went through testing to find out if something was wrong. After being informed that we couldn't have children, we decided to adopt. Our first son, David, arrived in 1985, and we planned to adopt another little boy, Graham, in 1988. We later realized that it may well have been the same week that we brought Graham home that Nancy became pregnant! After years of frustration and disappointment, the unexpected news of my wife's pregnancy came as a special joy for us. Under the circumstances, the possibility of my being diagnosed with a life-threatening disease was simply unimaginable.

That summer Nancy gave birth to our beautiful daughter, Whitney. Ironically, this undeniable proof that I was fertile led Nancy to suggest that I have a vasectomy. On my wife's birthday, November 10th, I went to a local urologist and had the operation. That night we had some friends over

---

for a birthday party. We were elated with our recent good fortune, and the evening was highlighted by a mock vasectomy performed behind a backlit screen—Happy birthday, Honey! Of course, it never occurred to us that our lighthearted antics might have been tempting fate.

A couple of months later I noticed a little blood in my urine. Although I felt no pain or discomfort, I immediately called the urologist who had performed my vasectomy. The doctor suspected that it was an infection from the operation and prescribed some antibiotics for me. After two weeks went by and the problem still hadn't cleared up, I went in to see the doctor, and he performed an ultrasound. From what I could make out, the images on the screen could have been anything from the air traffic at O'Hare to an old monochrome video game. But almost immediately, the doctor detected a spot on my prostate, and pointed it out for me. It appeared as a hazy bright patch on the screen, about the size of a dime.

The doctor later performed a biopsy, guiding a needle probe with the ultrasound to take samples from my prostate. The probe didn't hurt particularly. I know that many men suffer considerable anxiety and stress over these tests, whether it be from the invasion or associated discomfort. But these procedures really take less of a toll on us than we imagine. Much of the distress is psychological rather than physical. After a while, most patients become accustomed to the routine, and it all becomes very matter of course.

After my first round of tests, I went home feeling somewhat relieved. The spot on my prostate was a bit disturbing at first, but I really didn't think too much about it. The doctor hadn't said much during the biopsy, and afterwards, he didn't seem overly concerned. He told me that he would be sending the samples to a lab for examination, and would get back to me with the results in about ten days. I went back to my business as usual and thought no more about it.

Ten days later, the call came to my office. Rather than tell me the results of the biopsy over the phone, the doctor wanted to see me in person. That was my first inkling that something had to be wrong. I dropped by the urologist's office, not knowing what to expect. I was directed to wait in a small room, and the doctor soon came in with the results of my biopsy in a folder. He didn't look at me, but instead kept his eyes on his watch, as though pressed for time. In a matter-of-fact tone, he said, "You've got prostate cancer, and we have to operate. We can give you a penile implant."

I was totally dumbstruck. What little else the doctor told me I remember only vaguely. The diagnosis came as an overwhelming shock. I had cancer! The "big C." I was told I would have to return for some additional tests to see how far the cancer had spread. My mind was in a fog. I nodded dumbly. I couldn't even think clearly enough to ask any questions about my condition. I walked out of the office with nothing, not even a brochure.

I had been told I had prostate cancer, but that meant nothing to me. All I knew was what we all know, that cancer kills. Most of us have some notion of how our lives are going to play out. While we may not know exactly what cards we'll be dealt, we usually have some image of the future. But the realization that I had cancer had in one moment eclipsed the sense I had of my own bright future and threatened to blot out the life I had envisioned for myself.

That evening I went to my racquetball club and pounded a ball off the wall. What was happening was inconceivable. I was still young. I had a beautiful wife and three young children, two of them still in diapers. The words of an associate flashed into my mind. He once told me that he had lost his father when he was four. Were my children going to grow up without a father?

What made the situation all the more maddening was that I felt fine. As I stood there pounding on the racquetball, it seemed to me that I was as healthy as ever. How could I possibly be dying? I wondered if somehow a mistake had been made. A misdiagnosis. A slip-up at the lab. Something. I was grasping for straws, and my mind was reeling out of control. I had always been a strong, resourceful man, a tenacious problem solver, but suddenly I was confronted with this nightmare that went beyond anything I had ever had to face.

For the next few days, I didn't tell anyone about my secret. Not my friends, not my legal associates, not even my wife. I was still in shock and felt I needed some time to come to grips with the situation on my own. I threw myself into my work. Construction on my law office was near completion, and when I wasn't involved with a client, I kept myself occupied with the selection of carpets and wallpaper, colors and furnishings for the various rooms. The work was therapeutic, and at least to some degree allowed me to turn my attention to things other than my recent diagnosis.

But in the back of my mind, the problem continued to grind away. At moments, the nagging feeling would overcome me and I would find myself tormented by questions about what my condition meant and what the future held for me. Members of my staff, who were like a family to me, noticed that I was very quiet and withdrawn. Eventually, one of my secretaries came into my office and asked me if there was something wrong. I didn't even want to say the word—I simply told her that I had the big C.

At the end of the week, I decided to tell Nancy. Intellectually, I realized that she had a right to know, since this problem would deeply affect her as well. But emotionally up until that point, I hadn't been capable of sharing the painful reality of my diagnosis. Knowing that I had an appointment to see the urologist for follow-up tests within a few days, I now wanted her to go with me. My wife is very supportive, and I knew, whatever happened, that I could depend on her.

Of course, my wife had been aware all along that something was wrong. I was morose and incommunicative, not at all my normal self. There had been occasions in the past when my concerns at work weighed on me at home, but never quite so visibly. Because I prefer to solve work-related difficulties on my own, Nancy had chosen to wait until I was ready to tell her what was bothering me. She would later tell me that I was more depressed than she had ever seen me.

When the moment of truth finally arrived, I didn't know what to say to her. I just mumbled, "I've got prostate cancer," and left it at that. Nancy was clearly concerned, but took the news with characteristic quiet strength, bravely expressing her confidence that we would get through this calamity. Just knowing she knew relieved some of the psychological burden immediately. Having been consumed with doubts and fears, it was now a great comfort to know that I wasn't alone.

Normally, my wife would call close friends and family when she needed someone to talk to, but I asked her to keep it to herself for a while. She found it very difficult to hold in such a momentous revelation, but for my sake, she agreed. I wasn't ready for the world to know about my condition, but after a week of emotional paralysis, I was closer to being able to take action. We went to a bookstore and started doing our own research on prostate cancer.

The Search for Answers

The ensuing months would be taken up with relentless searching. I gathered as much material as I could find on the subject. I read and reread what I found, trying to make sense of it all. Each article, newspaper clipping and pamphlet was like a piece to a complex puzzle. I could only hope that when I finally put all the pieces together, I would know what I had to do.

In March of 1990, Nancy accompanied me when I returned to the urologist for various work-up tests, including a bone scan and CT scan. At the time, the PSA blood test was not yet being used as widely as it is today, when most men my age are as familiar with their PSA and its fluctuations as they are with their golf scores. I didn't have my PSA tested until after I had undergone treatment.

About a week after my follow-up tests, my wife and I met with the doctor to discuss the results. As before, he was brief and appeared hurried. He indicated that the tests showed no spread of the cancer beyond the prostate. I had been clinically diagnosed with what was then called stage B2 prostate cancer (what would now be termed stage T2c), the latest stage of prostate cancer still confined to the gland. It was still curable, but only if I acted in time. Once again, he strongly urged to have the cancer cut out as soon as possible.

I was relieved to hear the cancer was still contained, but I still didn't feel I knew enough about my condition to make an informed decision. He explained that I would be in the hospital for seven to ten days and laid up for another six to eight weeks. The doctor impressed upon me the urgency of my situation by saying that I needed to have the operation before the cancer spread any further. That scared me. But the potential consequences of the procedure were also frightening. I would probably be impotent, and I might suffer from incontinence. I knew that a neighbor of mine recently had a radical prostatectomy and had almost died when he hemorrhaged on the operating table. He was now wearing diapers. I wasn't at all sure what to do.

One book I read suggested that any patient considering a major operation should obtain a second opinion. So I asked the doctor for a referral. "You can go to the Moffitt Cancer Center in Tampa," he told me. "But we're just as good as they are, and besides, we're closer."

After leaving his office, I still felt dissatisfied. Nancy is usually far more tolerant than I am, but she was even more displeased than I was with the doctor's manner. We decided that I should at least go to the Moffitt Center before making a final decision. A few days later, I spoke to a family doctor I knew. I told him about my condition and described how the urologist had pressured me to have the surgery. "Wow!" he said. "That seems a little severe of him, to insist on immediately cutting it out."

His statement confirmed my suspicions that I was being rushed into making a decision. "Where else can I go?" I asked. He recommended several medical centers, including Johns Hopkins in Baltimore. After some further consideration, I set up an appointment there. As a licensed pilot for many years, I planned to fly my own plane up to Baltimore. But first Nancy and I would visit the Moffitt Center in Tampa, which was only an hour's drive away from our home.

The Dilemma of Treatment Options

The director of the Moffitt Center spoke to us at length and provided us with additional information about the available methods of treatment. The director suggested two possible options in my case: external beam radiation therapy or radical surgery. He recommended the latter, because at that time surgery had a higher cure rate and was thought to be the Gold Standard for treating prostate cancer. He also informed me about the potential complications such as impotence and bladder control problems. But because of my age and early stage cancer, his prognosis was very favorable in my case. His optimism relieved some of my anxiety about the operation and its side effects, but I was still hoping to avoid or at least postpone such an ordeal.

I had been reading a prostate cancer handbook which suggested that one option for some patients was not to be treated, but rather to be monitored to see if the disease progresses to the point where some form of treatment is necessary. I asked the director if I might wait and postpone treatment for the time being. He listened thoughtfully, but pointed out that

I was still in my forties, and the cancer would in all likelihood continue to grow. It might be years before the cancer caused any further symptoms, but sooner or later the disease would catch up with me. "One day," he said, "You're going to hop off that plane of yours and your leg is going to break, because the cancer has gotten into your bones."

I realized at once that he was right. It would be irresponsible of me to wait and do nothing, and in the end I would suffer the consequences of my choice. I needed to take care of the problem before it was too late.

In early May, Nancy and I took off in my Piper Seneca to keep my appointment at Johns Hopkins. The weather was clear most of the flight, but we encountered a heavy cloud cover over Baltimore. The fog was as thick as pea soup all the way down on our approach to the airport, until we reached about 200 feet. Then we suddenly broke through and could see the landing strip stretched out before us. I hoped it was a good omen, that I might somehow break through the fog of my own uncertainty now that I had arrived in Baltimore.

I had good reason to be optimistic. By chance, that same week an article had appeared in *U.S. News & World Report* magazine (April 30, 1990) that rated the finest hospitals in the country. Doctors were surveyed to determine the best hospitals for each of twelve specialties. The article recommended that a man diagnosed with prostate cancer should seek care in a premier institution. I saw that Johns Hopkins had been selected by more doctors than any other hospital in the specialty of urology. Furthermore, the article mentioned a new nerve-sparing technique used in prostate surgery that reduced the likelihood of impotence. The procedure had been pioneered by Dr. Patrick Walsh, who was the chief of urology at Johns Hopkins. I began to think that there might be a happy resolution after all.

After we arrived at Johns Hopkins, we met with a third-year resident, who assisted Dr. Walsh in the urology department. "I know you're only here for a second opinion," he said. "But this is a great hospital." He suggested that instead of having the operation performed in Florida, I should be treated at Johns Hopkins. He made sense, but I was still reluctant. "You know," he continued. "You really should do something about this rather than just gather information and put it off. This operation will work for you."

He prevailed upon me to schedule an operation for August 6th, the earliest date available. Although Nancy would have supported me no matter what I chose to do, she seemed pleased that I was finally making a decision. The surgery appeared to be the most reasonable option, but I still harbored reservations. I felt healthy, and that puzzled me. Also, my neighbor's close call on the operating table and his post-operative problems came back to mind. If I could find a reasonable alternative, I was still secretly hoping to somehow avoid going through with the operation.

As we were preparing to leave, I asked the resident, "By the way, I had my medical reports sent up here. Have you gotten a look at them yet?"

"No," he replied.

"Well," I asked. "What makes you think I need to have this operation?"

He didn't really have an answer, and that troubled me.

It continued to trouble me even after I flew back to Florida and returned to work. Instead feeling confident that my problem would soon be taken care of, I was plagued by a new wave of doubts. All of the doctors I had seen were pushing me to have the operation. Each argued for his own reasons that I should have it done at his medical facility. The resident at Johns Hopkins had done the same, and without even looking at my test results! How could he have known what was in my best interest without evaluating my particular case?

Perhaps I'm just suspicious by nature, but it dawned on me that the resident may not have been serving my interests as much as the economic interests of the hospital, or perhaps his own desire to gain further surgical experience. I wanted to believe the doctors I had seen, but I wasn't convinced I had been told the whole truth. Did I know all the facts? Did I really know all my options? At this point in the journey, I wasn't sure who to trust, and returned home with serious misgivings.

The gray skies and chill winds of that winter of discontent, when I first learned I of my cancer, had given way to spring rains, green grass and blooming flowers. Everywhere, lizards scampered in the bright sunlight, and down by the water's edge near our house, trains of ducklings waddled single-file after their mothers. The season brought its recurrent gift of new life, light, and hope.

But little had changed for me.

I had returned from the fog-shrouded city of Baltimore with a date for my operation at Johns Hopkins. I had hoped for something more, something intangible. Peace, clarity, resolution. What I really longed for was a sense of closure to the agonizing dilemma of choosing a treatment, which seemingly came down to deciding between the least of evils.

In the days that followed, as I once again returned to work at my law practice, there remained niggling doubts about whether I was doing the right thing. Everything I had been told, everything I had learned, had pushed me toward my present path. The way seemed clear, and yet after all these months, something within me still resisted traveling down the path laid out for me. In my mind, one thought repeatedly asserted itself: Was a radical prostatectomy really the best course for me, or might there still be another, better way?

Finding the Road Less Traveled

At some point in my readings, I had come across the number for the National Cancer Institute's information line, 1-800-4-CANCER. Initially, I had been unable to get through and set the number aside. Finally, around the middle of May, I was able to reach one of the NCI representatives. I spoke with a woman named Maria. After informing her about the results of my biopsy and subsequent staging tests, I told her that I was already familiar with the conventional treatments for prostate cancer, but wanted to find out if there were any other options I might pursue.

Maria made it clear that she could not advise me concerning which treatment would be best for me, but she could tell me my alternatives. Then she asked me, given the stage of my cancer, what I understood my options to be. I said, "It looks like I have three choices: I can have a radical prostatectomy, external radiation therapy, or I can do nothing, which may not be the wisest choice, but at least it is another option. I guess that's about it."

"No, Mr. Kaltenbach," she said, "You have a fourth choice."

"Oh?"

She then told me about a new form of treatment called brachytherapy, which utilized radioactive seeds implanted directly into the prostate. At first I was disappointed. I had heard about seed implants before. From what I had been able to gather, major abdominal surgery was involved, and the results obtained with this treatment had not been particularly promising.

But Maria informed me this was a different approach. While there were as yet no long-term results available, the procedure had been greatly improved thanks to recent technological innovations and was now being performed on an outpatient basis, without cutting. She said this treatment, while still considered investigational at that point, was a real, viable alternative for patients with early stage prostate cancer. Suddenly, I was very excited.

As Maria described it to me, tiny titanium tubes filled with a radioactive isotope, either Palladium-103 or Iodine-125, are injected into the cancerous prostate. The seeds are visually guided into place with the aid of ultrasound, ensuring that the implants are accurately placed throughout the gland. Once implanted, the radiation within the seeds goes to work, killing the cancer. Designed to irradiate only the site of the cancer, seed implantation could deliver a much higher, cancer-killing dose of radiation than external beam radiation, and with fewer long-term complications.

Maria also informed me that although the new palladium implants, known as TheraSeeds, had only been in use for a few months, they appeared to offer some advantages over the Iodine-125 seed implants, which had been in use longer. I soon learned that Palladium has a half-life of only 17 days, and degrades rapidly compared with the 60 day half-life of radioactive iodine. Within six months, or about 10 half-lives, the palladium seeds become inert, and reside harmlessly within the prostate. In addition, the initial burst of radiation delivered by palladium is significantly higher, with lethal consequences for the cancer. Tumors are destroyed rapidly, with no time to recover. And because the effective range of radiation emitted by palladium seeds is only about a centimeter, the risk of damage to surrounding organs is minimized.

At a time when I was floundering, this news was a godsend. I thanked Maria and then called the manufacturer of the TheraSeed® implant, the Theragenics Corporation, located in Norcross, Georgia. They informed me that at the time there were only two cancer centers in the country performing the palladium seed implant procedure. One of them was the Georgia Prostate Center in Atlanta, founded and directed by Dr. Harold P. McDonald.

During the next week, I spoke to Dr. McDonald on several occasions. He was friendly and very professional. We discussed my condition at length, and he answered all of my questions with great patience. He also sent me a packet of information on the procedure. I was very encouraged by everything that I learned, but wanted to be certain I was making the right decision. As I began to develop a relationship with Dr. McDonald, I expressed my concerns to him. "I need to find a comfort level with this procedure. This is a new treatment, and I want to make sure that I won't be some sort of guinea pig. Would you mind if I spoke to some of your patients?"

He gave me the names of six of his patients, and I called them all. Each man who I spoke with raved about his treatment. One fellow was 41 years old, about my own age. He too had wished to avoid the risks of surgery and was completely satisfied with his choice to forgo the knife in favor of seeds. Only one of the men had experienced any difficulties. He had gone square dancing the weekend after being treated. After dancing, he had been very sore, and temporarily had to have a catheter put in. But what impressed me was that he felt well enough a couple days of after treatment to go square dancing. That was testimony to the ease of recovery following brachytherapy.

The enthusiasm of these men was infectious. As I listened to their stories, they described their struggle with the same concerns that I was experiencing: the desire to avoid the dangers of major surgery or external beam radiation, the fear of impotence and incontinence that often resulted from those conventional treatments, the hope for some better alternative. For each of these patients, the answer had been seeding, and I was beginning to believe it could be the answer for me as well.

With growing confidence, I called the McDonald clinic to find out what arrangements would be necessary if I chose to have the procedure done. I talked with one of the nurses on McDonald's staff, providing her with biographical information—details on my medical history, my insurance coverage, and so forth. While I was talking with her, we made a surprising discovery. Nine years earlier she had been living near my home in New Port Richey and had actually been a client of mine. In fact, at that time she had worked for the local urologist who had diagnosed my prostate cancer! It was one of those coincidences that seem almost providential.

There was really no point in delaying any longer. I now knew this was the right choice for me. I called Johns Hopkins and, with some relief, canceled my operation. Then I set a date for the seed implantation with the McDonald clinic. When I hung up the phone that last time, a feeling came over me that seemed almost unfamiliar with all the turmoil of recent months. It was peace of mind.

In and Out By Lunchtime

The day before the operation, Nancy and I flew up to Georgia. I needed a battery of tests done the day before, including an ultrasound and CT scan that were crucial for planning the procedure. It all seemed rather routine, and by now I was an old hand at test-taking.

The preoperative ultrasound and CT scan were particularly important. They are used to calculate the volume and position of the prostate in the body, an essential element of the preplanning stage of the procedure. I understood that the number of seeds implanted and the configuration of their placement vary according to the needs of each patient. Careful planning would ensure that the optimum level of radiation was administered to my prostate.

On the day of my procedure, I was admitted to the medical center a couple hours in advance. Three other men were to receive palladium seed implantation that same morning. I was to be the last.

Since the procedure was only minimally invasive, meaning there were no incisions to be made, I was given the option of receiving local or general anesthesia. I chose the local anesthetic, since it would give me the opportunity to talk on the intercom with Nancy, who would be watching on a TV monitor in an observation room.

When my time came, I was wheeled into the OR and placed on an operating table in what they call the "semi-lithotomy position," a fancy name that just means you are on your back with your legs up in stirrups. The nurses and other members of Dr. McDonald's team were all very professional, though I recall a couple of jokes in the OR about how it was "nice to see a man in stirrups for a change"—a sentiment no doubt shared by many woman, including my wife.

Once on the table, I was given the local anesthetic and prepped for the procedure. Cloth was draped over me to provide some measure of privacy. Then an abdominal catheter was then put in place to drain urine from the bladder during the operation. At that point, Dr. McDonald performed the implantation. Each needle was inserted into the prostate to a depth previously determined by the computerized treatment plan. Once in place, the tiny seeds appeared as rows of white dashes on the ultrasound monitor. 63 seeds later, it was all over. The entire operation was completed in less than an hour.

At around one o'clock, I was wheeled into a lounge and met by my wife. The anesthetic hadn't worn off, so my legs weren't working yet. Nancy and I met with the three other men who were treated that morning. They too were joined by their wives. At the doctor's suggestion, we had all brought sack lunches. So we sat together and ate and talked about the procedure. We were all in good spirits, and a jovial Dr. McDonald dropped in to chat with us for a few minutes before heading back to work.

A few hours later, I walked out of the Georgia Prostate Center into the bright Atlanta sunlight, carrying with me 63 radioactive seeds silently at work destroying my cancer. It boggled my mind to think that if not for a single phone call a couple of weeks earlier, I would surely have been undergoing major abdominal surgery and an extended hospital stay. Instead, after a routine check-up the next morning, I would be on my way home, and within a couple of days I could safely return to work. With the likelihood that I was cured and had a low risk of complications, I couldn't help but feel lucky.

The weekend after the operation, I was hiking with my kids in the mountains of North Carolina. Although it was now the second week of June, to me it seemed that spring had finally arrived.

Three months after my treatment, I returned to the McDonald clinic for my quarterly check-up. I was glad to see the friendly faces of Dr. McDonald and his staff. They had become like family to me. I was also anxious to find out if the treatment had worked. At that point, I was given a PSA test, followed by an ultrasound of the prostate. The blood test indicated my PSA level was at 1.3, well within the normal range. And the tumor in my prostate no longer showed up on ultrasound.

I was told that to all appearances, I was cancer-free.

Only someone who has gone through treatment for cancer can imagine the relief I felt at hearing the news. *The journey is finally over,* I said to myself. *My cancer is gone!* It seemed as though I had been lost and trying to find my way through some unknown land. With all my searching and with all the setbacks along the way, I had finally made it to my destination. I was cured. Now life could return to normal again.

Or so I thought.

"So when do I get my certificate declaring I am officially cured?" I asked Dr. McDonald after my third quarterly visit.

"I'm afraid I can't give you one of those." he said apologetically. "You're in remission now, but we can't guarantee the cancer won't return sometime in the future."

This was not the news I had been hoping for. The realization that I might never be, with absolute certainty, cured of my cancer was a hard blow to take. I wanted it to be all over. I wanted to drop the whole mess in the "Out" basket and have it all go away. Unfortunately, with prostate cancer, that isn't the way it works, regardless of which form of treatment a man chooses. All I could do was watch and wait, and hope for the best.

With every passing year, the odds increase in my favor that my cancer will not return. To check my progress, I was monitored with quarterly PSA testing the first year, then semi-annually for several years. Now I am tested annually with a PSA test and color-flow Doppler ultrasound So far, after more than fourteen years, I remain free of cancer. My PSA has stabilized at 0.1. Fortunately, I never had any incontinence except for a couple of weeks following the procedure when I experienced some mild urinary urgency.

Nor did I have any problems with potency. Which reminds me of a story. A few years after Nancy and I were married, we tried in earnest to have children. Soft music, candles, romantic dinners, cruises, and even boxer trunks. Often, I would get calls from Nancy at the office letting me know that her temperature was up and that I needed to come home as soon as possible! But nothing worked. So, as I've mentioned, we had the pleasure of adopting our two boys before Nancy gave birth to our daughter.

Now it was my turn. About six weeks after my seed implant procedure, I was feeling pretty frisky. Sex was on my mind morning, noon and night. In retrospect, my renewed sexual interest was probably a natural outcome of the relief that I was now on the backside of treatment and feeling terrific. I would call Nancy from the office and tell her, "I'm coming home as soon as possible. Please do get ready, dear."

I love paybacks!

A Mission of Hope

Some months after I was treated, I got a call from the local urologist who had diagnosed my cancer. He was the one who had first advised me to have a radical prostatectomy, and now he was curious to find out if I had had anything done for my prostate cancer. I told him that I had undergone palladium seed implantation.

"Oh, the McDonald clinic," he replied.

I hadn't mentioned the name of the clinic. It was apparent that he had known about the procedure all along. Why hadn't he told me about it?

This incident stuck in my mind. I wondered how many other men were being left in ignorance because their doctors failed to properly inform them about their options. After careful consideration, I eventually decided to go public about my experience with prostate cancer. I started speaking to various civic and support groups in the hope of helping others, and later I published my first book, *Prostate Cancer: A Survivor's Guide.* Over the years, my message has been simple: men who turn 40 should start having a prostate examination once a year; and those who are diagnosed with prostate cancer need to become informed about their treatment options before taking action.

Over the past ten years, rarely have I gone a day without receiving a call from someone with prostate cancer, or a relative or friend of a man with the disease. In many cases, my name came to them by word of mouth. Many of those who call have just been diagnosed and are terrified at what having prostate cancer might mean. I have seen men in their seventies struggle to hold back tears as they tell me about their diagnosis. Some men have been told by their doctors to undergo a particular treatment and want help finding a second opinion.

It never ceases to amaze me how little these men have been told. Many don't even know what stage of cancer they have. Nor are they usually familiar with their treatment options. In most cases, they have been left in the dark and are as desperate for information as I was.

During the past few years, the situation has improved, with most doctors at least providing a list of available primary treatment options. More information is available and the number of support groups around the country has multiplied dramatically. Yet many doctors remain biased toward treatments provided by their specialty. With surgery falling out of favor, some urologists engage in a kind of spin control, attempting to present the surgical option in the most favorable light, even to the extent of ignoring the most recent published data. Some doctors, aware of disagreements in the field concerning treatment options, may choose to shield their patients from controversy. When that occurs, the price to the patient is the loss of his freedom to choose.

Some doctors are reticent to admit they are not fully informed about a particular disease, yet family doctors and general practitioners may be unfamiliar with the latest and best treatments. No doubt there are some physicians who choose to keep their patients ignorant of the alternatives for fear of losing revenue. A great deal of misinformation continues to circulate. Whatever the reason, doctors often to fail to adequately inform their patients about their conditions and the treatments that are available. And all too often, patients are willing to relinquish their right to know the alternatives available to them, instead going on blind faith that the doctor knows what is best for them.

Unfortunately, the failure to fully disclose treatment options to the patient can lead to abuses. Anyone involved with prostate cancer patients hears his share of horror stories. I have talked to men in their seventies with stage T1 disease who have been told they have no recourse but to get a radical prostatectomy. Yet for most men in this age bracket, that early stage cancer will never pose a threat to the life of the patient. Unfortunately, this kind of abuse is still common. I remember hearing one prostate cancer researcher comment, "When surgeons are in doubt, they cut."

On the other hand, there are cases in which the physician treating a prostate cancer patient inexplicably waits when more immediate treatment would be appropriate. I remember one instance when a man in his sixties was diagnosed with early stage cancer and his doctor chose to simply monitor his PSA level. More than a year passed while his PSA steadily climbed, and his cancer progressed from its original early stage to meta-static disease. By that time, he had begun to experience symptoms and his chance for receiving curative treatment had been squandered.

I have also heard a number of stories from patients with advanced dis-ease whose urologists have advised them, "Cut it out and it will be gone." These patients were doomed to failure. Still more appalling, the urologist may say words to the effect, "If you were my father, I would advise you to have a radical prostatectomy." Sometimes he may add, "If you choose to have radiation therapy, I will cease to be your doctor." Unbelievable, but all very true.

Stories like these prompted me to establish the Prostate Cancer Re-source Foundation in 1996, to promote public awareness and to offer hope and encouragement for men with prostate cancer and their loved ones. As I found myself devoting more and more of my time to this mission over the next few years, I was happy to give up my law practice to help found and direct the Dattoli Cancer Center in the fall of 2000. With this career change, my journey with prostate cancer continues to this day, as a labor of love more gratifying than anything I had ever undertaken in my life.

As one who has experience as a prostate cancer patient and as a care-giver, my hope is that this book will arm men like myself with the knowl-edge to ask the right questions of their physicians, and with the necessary information to judge and evaluate the answers they receive. While my case history may be unique, there are challenges that all of us face when deal-ing with this disease. The emotional and financial aspects of the journey are areas that deserve special attention and they will be discussed in the pages immediately ahead.

CHAPTER TEN

THE EMOTIONAL BURDEN OF PROSTATE CANCER

The Traumatic Syndrome of Cancer

Although I didn't realize it at the time, the questions that I asked myself after my diagnosis reflected emotional reactions that anyone goes through after being diagnosed with cancer. The questions that we ask ourselves can tell us how we are coping with the emotional trauma of the disease and what psychological needs we need to address in order to carry on the fight. The following are some of the questions I found continually returning to my mind over the period of months before I was treated. In all likelihood, they will be familiar to any cancer patient.

"How can this be happening to me?"

The immediate reaction of anyone who learns they have cancer is most likely to be shock and disbelief. At first I felt as though the unimaginable had happened, like I'd been hit by a meteor. Often, this kind of reaction persists long after the discovery stage. Such feelings may surface again and again with the ups and downs of testing and treatment. Moments of panic and disbelief are normal and to be expected by anyone faced with cancer and its possible consequences. For men with prostate cancer, there is not only the threat of death, but the potential side effects of treatment that can seem almost as frightening as the disease.

The sense that your life is coming apart can leave you confused and unable to concentrate, or paralyzed and unable to act. The emotions that overtake us may seem strange and unnatural, but they are typical of anyone going through a traumatic experience. It is always a struggle to find a way to cope with the impact of disease. Underlying the question "How could this be happening to me?" and all the emotions that accompany it, we are really asking ourselves, "How do I make sense of this and cope with what has happened to me?" It is the first step in our struggle, a step we may need to retrace many times along the way. At times it may seem there is no answer to the question, but don't give up. When you feel panic, remind yourself of some important facts:

> Your body does not hate you. Life does not hate you. God does not hate you. You have a disease that needs to be treated.

> Prostate cancer is not synonymous with death. You have every reason to believe you will survive this ordeal.

> There are many available treatments to successfully combat the disease.

> There is no reason to expect permanent side effects, and if there are any, they can be controlled or mitigated.

> You can control the process of living with, treating, and overcoming your cancer.

> Cancer can open up positive avenues of change and growth in your life, whether they be emotional, relational or spiritual.

"How can I have cancer?"

I had always thought of cancer as a disease that afflicts the old, yet I was only in my early forties. I had three young children. How could I have cancer? The desire to avoid facing a painful truth can be overwhelming at times. We are in denial when our thoughts and perceptions don't conform to reality, but instead make attempts to escape from it. No matter how clear-headed a man may be, he is almost certain to experience some degree of denial after being confronted with the grim reality of cancer. Even doctors who have treated cancer patients may struggle with denial when they are themselves diagnosed with the disease.

Denial is a defense mechanism that allows us to avoid or block out information that we are psychologically unable to absorb all at once. This defense can manifest itself in a variety of ways. Frequently, a patient, when first informed of his cancer by his doctor, will fail to understand or later recall the details of his diagnosis. Some will avoid talking about the illness and pretend it doesn't exist. Still others will be unrealistically optimistic, refusing to accept the seriousness of their illness or expecting a sudden, miraculous cure. All of these reactions are symptomatic of denial.

Denial can be a blessing when it protects us from excessive anxiety or depression. A short vacation from a world of troubles can be a restorative for the mind and body. But reality has a way of catching up with those that run from it, and severe denial has a variety of harmful consequences. It may prevent a man from seeking proper medical treatment. Even if it doesn't interfere with his treatment, denial can distort his personal relationships and obstruct open and honest communication with friends and family members.

Most men who are diagnosed with prostate cancer will pass through a period of denial, and gradually come to an acceptance of their condition. In my case, many weeks passed before I surrendered my doubts about my diagnosis. I don't think I came to fully accept I had prostate cancer until being treated. Fortunately, these doubts did not interfere with my efforts to deal responsibly with the problem. I know of other men who were not so fortunate. I once heard about a local man who, after being diagnosed, refused to believe that he had prostate cancer. Time passed and eventually the disease spread throughout his body. He entered the latter stages of the disease and became terminal, but he still remained convinced that he had nothing but a bad case of the flu. It's okay to have doubts or suspicions about what a doctor tells you, but don't let it keep you from getting more information or finding medical care. Your life may depend on it.

"Why me?"

After the initial shock of diagnosis, most patients experience some form of depression. Weeping, despair, and a sense of guilt are all symptoms of depression and are completely normal. Men often feel that tears are a sign of weakness, or that we should be tough and stand up to adversity, rather than succumb to grief. But who would say to someone who is overcome at the loss of a loved one, "Buck up! Be a man and stop your moping!" The prospects confronting a cancer patient can seem far worse: the loss of life and loved ones and everything he cherishes.

It is understandable that a man should become depressed with the prospect of such losses. If you have prostate cancer, don't punish yourself for feeling down. The support of those who care about you can be a comfort. Prayer or meditation can also lift your spirits. If you know someone who has the disease and is gripped by depression, you need not always try to cheer him up or talk him out of being sad. It is often enough simply to be there for that person in order to offer sympathetic understanding of what he is going through.

"Will I lose my family? "

Losing my family was my greatest fear, even greater than the fear of death. The idea that my children might grow up without their father tormented me. As in my case, the fear of death for many men is often accompanied or overshadowed by other fears and anxieties. Among them are: fear of pain, fear of impairment or humiliation, fear of being a burden, fear of being alone or deserted, and fear of financial difficulties due to the costs of medical treatment.

Such crises elicit in us a myriad of fears and inadequacies that would otherwise remain at bay. These added insecurities can weigh us down and magnify the stress we feel as we seek to manage not only our cancer but its impact on every aspect of our lives. At times the burden may seem too much to bear, so don't try to bear it all on your own. Rely on the support of family and friends, and share your concerns with them. You may find it helpful to turn to your local church for spiritual guidance and financial aid. Hospitals often provide counseling for cancer outpatients in need of emotional support. And as mentioned, there are also a number of support groups for men with prostate cancer and their families *(see Appendix B: Where To Get Help)*.

In the midst of this crisis, it is important that you not dwell on your problems to such an extent that they leave you feeling helpless. You are not helpless. Determine what actions you can take on your own behalf, and set realistic goals for yourself. Only you can take responsibility for directing your cancer treatment, so become informed, seek out good medical care, and look after your health.

By keeping yourself active, you can avoid fixating on your problems. Work and exercise were both helpful to me in keeping a sense of order to life and taking my mind off my problems. If you still work, make it business as usual as best you can. Social activities can serve as a valuable outlet as well. At times you may not feel like doing any of these things, but your emotional well-being has an impact on your health. It may help if you look at these areas as being part of your medical treatment.

"How can anyone know what I'm going through?"

Most cancer patients experience some degree of isolation as a consequence of their disease. Many report feeling separated from the world or different from others. The reality of the illness becomes an invisible barrier between the sufferer and other people.

There are two causes for this sense of isolation. The first comes from within the person suffering from cancer. The flood of internal feelings and emotions may act to drive him away from others. He may feel strange, uncomfortable or embarrassed in their presence. He may withdraw and wish only be alone. I know that when something is bothering me, I have a tendency to become quiet and withdraw into myself. It's a common reaction.

The other cause of isolation works from the outside: the social stigma attached to cancer or any serious illness. Our culture prizes health and well-being, and displays an unnatural fear of illness and death. We keep sick people in hospitals, away from the rest of society, thus enabling us to avoid the difficult issues of sickness and mortality. It may be as others have suggested that our whole society is in denial over death.

Our cultural biases are reflected in our attitudes toward the sick. We often don't know what to say or how to act around the sick person, and feel discomfort being near him or her. Even loved ones may respond this way. Many avoid the sick person, in part perhaps because he or she is a reminder that cancer can strike anyone. They turn a blind eye to the illness and tell themselves. "It can't happen to me."

Before my cancer experience, I would hear about someone who had the disease and say that it was a shame. Although I could express sympathy for others with cancer, I didn't really know how to relate to them or their ordeal. You have to go through it yourself, and once you do, your eyes are opened. Cancer suddenly becomes real and personal to you, and then you understand just how they felt. I suspect that most people are like I was before my diagnosis. Until they have felt the personal impact of cancer on their own lives, they will not be able to truly identify with your situation.

The Emotinal Course of Prostate Cancer

1. Initial Diagnosis often involves anxiety and distress. This early phase can also cause sadness and depressed moods, loss of sleep or oversleeping, fatigue, decreased libido, confusion, difficulty making decisions, restlessness, irritability, weight loss and anorexia.

2. Treatment Planning often alleviates anxiety and distress as the patient begins to learn about the disease and weigh treatment options. Once the patient has decided on a course of treatment, there is usually a sense of relief and improved mental outlook.

3. Treatment Initiation or the immediate anticipation of treatment may cause a brief increase in anxiety and distress, but usually not as severe as experienced at the time of initial diagnosis.

4. Treatment Adaptation takes place in the period following treatment, as the patient learns to cope with his therapy and any side effects he may experience. Successful therapy will usually bring about a reduction of anxiety and distress, while complications or an unfavorable outcome can lead to further emotional distress. When a patient's mood does not improve after being successfully treated, it may be a sign of clinical depression that needs to be addressed.

You may sense that people treat you differently, which can intensify your sense of isolation and leave you feeling alone in your fight against the disease. If you feel isolated, find someone you can trust to open up and express how you're feeling. This may be a family member, friend, counselor, or someone else who has had the disease.

These are only a few of the questions that men who have prostate cancer will ask themselves. Behind the questions are a seething host of powerful emotions: fear, anger, confusion, self-pity, bitterness, despair, and others. Doctors can help the body in its battle against the cancer, but they can do little to help the patient in his fight to come to grips with the emotional and psychological impacts of prostate cancer. Yet at the same time, there is a growing awareness in the medical community of the important role the patient's emotions have in his recovery. Negative emotions can weaken the immune system, but a positive attitude can aid it in its fight.

Thus, in a sense half the battle is up to you. Although a positive mental attitude in and of itself cannot cure you, it can enhance the body's response to treatment. But don't think if you do have periods of anxiety, anger, or depression that you have failed, or are somehow "making yourself worse." Anyone who suffers from cancer will struggle with these feelings from time to time. The important thing is to not succumb to them.

Opposite these negative emotions are positive emotions and attitudes that can strengthen you. Courage, confidence, amusement, serenity, joy in the little things in life, and, above all, hope. Cultivate these. They are the best weapons we have in our battle against this disease.

Treating Clinical Depression

As mentioned, a prostate cancer diagnosis often brings feelings of sorrow, fear and desperation. When these feelings are prolonged, they may be indicative of a more serious clinical depression. Studies have shown that as many as 20% of cancer patients suffer from clinical depression, which involves persistent depressive symptoms, such as hopelessness, despair, and pervasive thoughts of suicide and death. There may also be physical symptoms such as loss of appetite and insomnia. A diagnosis of depression based on these physical symptoms is problematic because these same symptoms may be due to the cancer itself or they may be side effects of various cancer therapies such as hormonal therapy. Recent studies have shown that proteins called cytokines, which may be produced by the tumor or by an immunological response to the tumor, can cause psychological symptoms such as depression and anxiety.

It may be difficult for some patients to ask for help, but it's not necessary to suffer in silence. Clinical depression is a treatable disease, and the first step in getting help is to alert your doctor or other healthcare practi-

SURVIVING PROSTATE CANCER WITHOUT SURGERY

tioner that you are experiencing symptoms. The National Comprehensive Cancer Network (NCCN, www.nccn.org) has developed specific guidelines to help practitioners screen for depression on a case by case basis. Patients suffering from clinical depression are often referred to a mental health professional, such as a psychiatrist or psychologist, who can assess what type of treatment may be warranted.

Typically, the same anti-depressant drugs are used to treat clinical depression in cancer patients as those used to treat otherwise healthy patients. Studies have shown that cancer patients who experience clinical depression are highly responsive to anti-depressant treatment. For patients with mild to moderate depression, psychotherapy alone may be enough. For patients with moderate to severe depression, both psychotherapy and medication are often utilized. A wide range of anti-depressant drugs are available. They vary considerably as far as their side effects, safety and tolerability, and patients are advised to discuss the advantages and disadvantages of specific anti-depressant medications with their doctors.

Some of the newer anti-depressant medications such as the group known as selective seratonin uptake inhibitors (SSRIs) tend to have milder side effects and are easier to tolerate than some of the older drugs. The SSRIs include Prozac®, Zoloft®, Paxil®, Celexa®, and Lexapro®. Their side effects can include headaches, difficulty sleeping, stomach distress and decreased libido. It should be emphasized that depression is a disease just like prostate cancer is a disease, and both are treatable with modern therapies.

When Your Husband or Significant Other has Prostate Cancer

Looking back, that very first week after I was diagnosed is still vivid in my mind. It was the longest, hardest, and loneliest week I ever went through. Those were the seven days that I withheld my terrible secret from everyone, including the person closest to me, my wife. After I confided in Nancy, some of my emotional turmoil was alleviated, but for her the crisis was just beginning. With the fallout of diagnosis still clouding my mind, my own problems dominated my thoughts. It occurred to me, after all, she wasn't the one who had been diagnosed with cancer.

There is a common misconception that with cancer there is only one real casualty. But in fact, those who are close to a patient may be vicarious victims. Like most spouses, Nancy also assumed that because I was the one with cancer, I was the one in need of love and support. This same attitude is mirrored to some extent by healthcare providers, who tend to focus, sometimes exclusively, on the problems of the cancer patient. After all, the patient is the most obvious victim.

In the traditional view of the medical community and its support services, the nuclear family is seen primarily as a source of emotional support to those facing cancer. Of course, the person with the disease is the only one who faces bodily harm caused by cancer, and that ultimate of physical consequences, death. And certainly those closest to the patient can be of great value in providing him with comfort and support. But this should not lead us to diminish the cost to others. The devastation wrought by cancer does not stop with the cancer patient. It spreads to spouses, relatives, friends—in essence, everyone who knows and cares for the cancer sufferer. To a greater or lesser degree, they are all victims of the disease. Of course, those closest to the cancer patient, physically and emotionally, are likely to suffer the greatest repercussions.

For a man with prostate cancer, there is usually one other principal victim of the disease: his wife or significant other. Prostate cancer can turn her life upside down much as his own. Children too—especially when young and still dependent on their parents—can be greatly victimized by their father's cancer. The emotional cost to them can be enormous. But parents are often able to act as a buffer between their children and the full impact of the disease. The man and his wife who find ways to bear the brunt of the burden together can help to minimize the impact of the disease on their kids. Because prostate cancer usually strikes men over the age of 60, in the majority of cases the children will be grown and out of the house. This doesn't mean they won't be affected. But separate lives and separate addresses are likely to shield them to some extent, leaving only the man with prostate cancer and his spouse to suffer the full impact of the disease.

For a wife, although there is no tumor within her body, her husband's prostate cancer does have a real and palpable presence in her life. Because of it, she too must face tormenting questions: Will my husband die? Will my children lose their father? How will I live without him? How will I make ends meet? What can I do? And like her husband, she will at times undoubtedly wonder, Why me?

Her daily life will be irrevocably changed. Her accustomed duties and activities may be completely disrupted. She may find herself weighed down with new and unfamiliar responsibilities, as she faces the prospect of caring for and possibly supporting her husband during and after his treatment. With her husband, she must cope with the impact that the disease may have on their marriage relationship—their sex life, their social life, and the way they interact together may all be dramatically altered. In so many ways, she is a partner to his pain.

Coping with the Pains Of Partnership

If your husband or significant other has prostate cancer, then you already have firsthand experience with the pains of partnership. While men typically go through a variety of emotional conflicts when confronted with cancer, you too must endure the emotional turmoil that has come about as a consequence of his disease. Although you may be experiencing emotions similar to those of your husband, you are likely to have other problems to deal with that are unique. How can you cope with your own feelings and emotions while providing support and encouragement to your husband?

This is the paradox you must find a way to resolve as the partner of a prostate cancer patient. Although you may suffer from the ravages of your husband's cancer as intensely as he does, you also find yourself thrust into the role of caretaker. In an effort to ease your husband's suffering, you may choose, as many wives do, to suffer in silence while making every effort to appear cheerful and optimistic. This approach may work occasionally, but often it will backfire. He may sense that you are not being open with him or treating him as an adult, which will only add to his feelings of isolation and helplessness. Furthermore, maintaining the facade can place additional strains on your relationship, sometimes leading to increased conflict or even breakdown.

The well-being of your marriage may depend on finding a balance between your own emotional needs and the physical and emotional needs of your husband. Like all troubles that couples face in life, the battle against prostate cancer is best undertaken as a partnership. Both you and your husband will be better off if you can work together as a team against the common enemy. It is important to be aware of the emotions and related psychological problems that you may have to confront as a consequence of your husband's prostate cancer.

Keeping Fears Under Control

Cancer is always very frightening. Even the word is scary. Because you have almost as much to lose as your spouse, it is to be expected that you will suffer a great deal of fear and anxiety. The idea of losing your loved one may be overwhelming. And your husband's fears may intensify your own distress.

Sometimes the increased demands placed on you can be frightening, especially in the face of an uncertain future. You may feel inadequate to deal with all of your new responsibilities. Worrying over your husband's condition may leave you troubled and distraught, anxious and uncertain about how to help him and yourself during this crisis. Confusion, moments of panic, and interrupted sleep patterns can all result from such chronic anxiety.

Fears are normal and unavoidable when cancer is involved. But if you find yourself struggling to keep your fears under control, there are some things you can do to make your anxieties more manageable:

Remember that prostate cancer is usually slow growing.

Most men with prostate cancer do not die of the disease, and will usually live for years after diagnosis. You have time yet to be together. Making an effort to learn more about the disease and its treatment may help to allay your fears.

Be aware that worrying won't make your husband or partner any better.

Excessive concern may cause you to become overprotective or even smothering. Or you may find yourself "walking on pins and needles" to avoid doing anything to upset your husband. Although these behaviors are intended to relieve the strains your husband is going through, usually they will only add to them. On the other hand, indiscriminately pouring out all your anxieties on your husband is an unnecessary burden for him to bear. He has plenty of fears of his own. Try to treat him much as you normally would, but don't be afraid to gently express your concern for him. In this way, you can be a comfort to him, and hopefully he will respond in a way that will help to comfort your fears.

Share your fears and concerns with others.

Merely talking to family members was a relief for my wife. Simply knowing she didn't have to deal with her fears alone helped to alleviate them. Be cautious however with any family member you think may be unable to handle the news. Young children especially should not be overburdened with your fears since they are usually less able to deal with them.

Join a support group.

Like your husband, you may benefit from joining a support group. Man To Man and US TOO!™ are both dedicated specifically to prostate cancer patients and their families (see Appendix B: Where To Get Help). Sympathetic strangers who understand what you are going through can be a great source of comfort without the potential complications that can arise when family and friends are involved.

Keep yourself active.

Do things to take your mind off your troubles. If you find yourself attending to your husband and his needs to the exclusion of all else, you might find some way to get away for a while. It will do both of you good.

Practice relaxation techniques.

Many people can help to reduce their tension level through the use of breathing exercises, progressive relaxation, meditation, and other relaxation techniques.

Pray.

People with spiritual convictions find solace through prayer. Nancy and I found our faith to be a source of comfort and strength during the darkest hours.

Take one day at a time.

Resist the urge to become fixated on what the unknowable future may hold. Take reasonable steps to prepare for any contingency, but keep your mind focused on the short-term. Similarly, keep your thoughts on those things over which you have some control, rather than things you cannot control, such as the results of your husband's diagnostic tests. In this way, you can maximize the help you can provide to your family while minimizing your anxieties.

Defusing Anger and Resentment

If you have experienced feelings of irrational anger directed at your husband since his diagnosis with prostate cancer, you are not the only one. Anger is an emotion that you may have difficulty admitting to yourself or expressing to others. Our society seems to regard anger as an inappropriate emotion in women, and many women tend to repress such feelings. The discomfort that many women experience in this regard may be especially unsettling under circumstances such as these, when any negative feelings seem so inappropriate.

Do you find your temper flaring up unexpectedly, or feel a growing sense of resentment toward your husband? Perhaps it makes you feel guilty or ashamed to resent your husband in his hour of need. You may be telling yourself that it isn't really his fault that he's sick, but feelings of resentment are a natural reaction to the additional frustrations of your situation.

You may be longing for the way things were. But now, new duties, greater demands on your time, and yearnings that are frustrated are likely to increase the stress of your daily life. He may not be doing what you think is necessary. Feelings of anger are likely to arise with increased tensions.

Coping with anger isn't easy, but it can be done. The first hurdle is to admit to yourself that you really are angry. An inability to acknowledge the anger can lead to far more destructive behavior. You may begin to feel more distant and indifferent toward your husband. You may turn on others besides your husband, or you may become deeply depressed and self-destructive. Far better than any of these reactions is facing your anger honestly and finding ways to overcome it.

To defuse your anger, recognize that its source is the increased stress of the situation, not your spouse. If you have been having conflicts with your husband, he too may be dealing with anger arising from frustration over his condition. Perhaps he is feeling helpless and dependent, and taking it out on you. Knowing this, direct your anger at the real source of frustration for both of you: the cancer itself. The best way to beat the enemy is to take the lead in supporting your husband.

At the same time, find ways to release tension and frustration. Do something that you enjoy. Go shopping, see a movie, visit a friend. Anything that reduces pent up stress will help you control feelings of anger. Crying is one common and effective way women sublimate feelings of anger they wish to avoid expressing in a more destructive way. Tears can be therapeutic and stress-reducing. But keep in mind that although a good cry may be a wonderful release for you, your husband might find it very upsetting. Try to find someplace away from him for your tears, so that you don't increase his stress while reducing your own.

You may feel that your anger is justified. Perhaps you feel you are bearing too much of the burden for your husband. If so, try to avoid venting your anger on him. Instead, talk with him as calmly and gently as you can (see Opening the Lines of Communication below). Remember what he is going through as well when you find yourself struggling to control your temper. You need support for yourself, too, so don't be ashamed to accept help from friends and family to relieve some of your burden.

Overcoming Feelings of Guilt

Feelings of guilt may accompany thoughts of failure and self-blame. Perhaps you feel you are not doing enough for your partner, or that you are failing to live up to your obligations. Do you feel a sudden aversion to your loved one now that he has been diagnosed with cancer? Do you find yourself trying to avoid spending time with him? Resentment of your husband or the limitations that his disease has imposed on your life may leave you feeling like a neglectful wife. Perhaps you feel ashamed of inappropriate thoughts that have come unexpectedly to your mind. You may even be blaming yourself for your husband's illness.

All of these things can instill a sense of guilt. You might ask yourself what is at the root of your feelings of guilt. Have you done anything for which your conscience is bothering you? Are your guilty feelings exaggerated? You may have unrealistic expectations of yourself, in which case you need to come to an understanding of what you can and cannot do. One thing you cannot do is make your husband better, any more than you could have prevented his prostate cancer in the first place. Your love and support is important to your husband, but your constant attention is probably unwarranted. Indeed, he may be feeling guilty for the demands his condition is placing on you. For both your sakes, try to find a happy medium between caring for your husband and taking care of your own well-being.

As mentioned, many people experience aversion around sick individuals. If you do, remind yourself that although he is ill, your husband is the same man he always was. If his body has been affected by the disease, his spirit remains unchanged. Also keep in mind that his cancer is not contagious and cannot harm you in any way. Use your desire to be supportive as a weapon against these irrational feelings of aversion and the guilt they produce.

If you conclude that you have real reason to feel guilty, do something about it. Escape and avoidance are common but largely unproductive coping responses. If you respond to pressure by looking for an escape route, work on changing your response. Also seek ways to reduce the amount of pressure you feel. Even guilt can be used as an escape, so don't dwell on your guilt feelings. Instead, take positive actions to lessen the guilt you feel. Don't allow yourself to get caught in an endless cycle of failure and self-condemnation. If you feel like running away, try setting limited short-term goals that you feel confident you can accomplish.

Dealing with Depression

Some degree of depression may be unavoidable. It's to be expected. Along with your husband, you may experience many ups and downs during his treatment for prostate cancer. But when a period of discouragement slides into chronic depression, real problems can result. For this reason, it is important to overcome these natural periods of melancholy and despondency if they show signs of persisting.

Depression can have a wide range of effects. You may feel listless or exhausted, and unable to enjoy the things that normally bring you pleasure.

Interacting with others may become a chore, and your daily tasks may suddenly seem too much to bear. Perhaps the idea of your loved one's suffering and possible loss may be unutterably depressing to you. Changes in your life—difficult adjustments and altered plans—may come as disappointments. And because prostate cancer can be a long-term problem, stretching into years, hopelessness may set in, threatening an even deeper and more persistent state of despair.

Your depression may stem from an inability to express your true feelings. The drain of always trying to maintain a cheerful face for your husband's sake may be fueling your feelings of depression. Your attempts to steadfastly maintain a positive demeanor are not only unrealistic but may not be responsive to your husband's real needs. If he is sad and depressed, your apparent cheerfulness may leave him feeling isolated. He may even feel you don't really care about what is happening to him. But in reality, grief is often love experiencing loss. Sharing your sorrows and grief together over your mutual losses can be an expression of love, and may provide a bridge out of despair for both of you.

Exerting the necessary effort to overcome your depression can sometimes seem depressing in and of itself! But it's worth it. Examine yourself to see if any of the negative emotions described above are contributing to your depression. If so, take what steps you can to control those emotions. When feelings of sorrow, despair and anxiety persist over weeks and months, clinical depression may be indicated. Wives and partners who feel they may be experiencing symptoms of clinical depression are advised to communicate their concerns to their doctors and to keep in mind the guidelines for care discussed earlier in this chapter (see Treating Clinical Depression).

Opening the Lines of Communication

Many patients learn the importance of open communication in establishing a relationship of trust with their doctors. Similarly, honest and open expression between you and your husband is needed if the two of you are to successfully turn the resources of your marriage to solving the problems you confront. In the same way that a failure to be forthcoming can undermine the doctor-patient relationship, an atmosphere of secrecy can develop within a family or marriage when information is withheld from the patient "for his own good."

The emotionally charged issues generated by prostate cancer can be difficult to talk about. A couple who have always maintained honest, intimate communication in their relationship may find that the disease has created a wall of silence between them. Many marriages have never achieved the level of open communication that this situation demands of them. For these couples, the very idea of expressing the complex emotions they are experiencing may seem unimaginable.

Often each partner is afraid to say anything that might hurt the other. They try to protect each other by hiding the emotions they are feeling. It may seem easier and more comfortable that way, but at a time when they need each other most, a pattern of withholding leads both into isolation. This can intensify their negative emotions and lead to exaggerated fears about what his or her partner is going through.

In such an atmosphere, both partners may come to feel as though they are living with a monster in their midst, yet are compelled to ignore its existence. The lack of communication between them undermines their ability to show love and support for each other. Only by bridging the gulf between them can their relationship contribute to healing and harmony.

Not everyone is able to express disturbing emotions, or talk about the frightening life-changes that emerge from a serious illness. No one should be compelled to talk against his or her will. There is no guarantee that every couple will successfully cope with all the new pressures on their relationship. The strain on some relationships can result in divisions in the marriage and professional counseling may be needed to save the relationship. But those couples that grow closer and stronger in such a crisis usually do so by striving to maintain honest and open communication.

When It's Time To Talk

The first steps toward openness can be the most difficult, even terrifying. No matter how well you know your husband, you are unlikely to know for sure how he will react. You may be afraid of losing control of your own emotions should you open up. Perhaps you simply don't know how to begin such a momentous conversation.

There is no easy set of rules to follow to develop good communication. People and their relationships differ. You will have to rely on a certain degree of intuition to know when is a good time for the two of you to talk.

Here are a few guidelines that may make it a little easier to open the lines of communication with your spouse or partner.

Give him time to adjust.

Every man has his own emotional timetable for coming to terms with the impact of cancer. Like me, your husband may need a period of private introspection. Respect his privacy rather than trying to push him into a discussion of his illness before he is ready. You too will probably need time to recover your emotional equilibrium. It's not uncommon for the spouse of a prostate cancer sufferer to have a more difficult time coping with the disease than the patient himself does.

If you are having a hard time absorbing the shock of your partner's diagnosis, you may not feel ready to talk. You may be having trouble accepting the situation. If so, try not to shut him out or avoid him if he seeks to talk seriously with you. After all, it probably took considerable courage for him to risk initiating conversation about this sensitive issue. Express a willingness to talk with him, but request that he give you a little more time to digest the news. You might suggest a day sometime in the near future when you will be ready to talk.

Be prepared to share your concerns.

Try to put your feelings into words before talking with your husband. Do you identify with any of the emotional responses described in the previous sections? What are your concerns about his prostate cancer and its treatment? What questions do you have about what your husband is feeling or what you can do for him?

It may help you to clarify your concerns by writing down those things you would like to talk about with your partner. Talking through your feelings with someone else first may also help. This person could be a friend, family member, or professional counselor. Or you might want to talk to someone who can better identify with your situation. As indicated previously, there are support groups and cancer hotlines that will allow you to speak directly to others who have experienced the disease firsthand (see

Appendix B: Where To Get Help). Don't hesitate to reach out when you need help.

Let him choose the time to talk.

Your husband is the one most intimately affected by the cancer. For this reason, allow him to choose the moment to initiate discussion about his condition. The first words may be halting and brief—he may not say much at all—but that's all right. After all, you don't need to say everything immediately. Some things you may never need to say. What is most important is that the door will have been opened.

In the meantime, you don't have to wait idly for your husband to break the silence. There are ways you can encourage openness. Indicate a readiness to listen, and show your support for him through your attention to his needs. A touch, a hug, a loving gesture will let him know you are there for him. That way, when he is ready to talk, he will know that you have a willing and sympathetic ear waiting for him.

Look for cues.

Just like you, your husband may not know how to begin. Watch for signs that he wants to talk, but is struggling to find the words. If you are usually the verbal initiator in your marriage relationship, he may be waiting for you to start. Awkwardness or nervousness in your presence, or talking around the subject, are often good indications that he wants to talk openly. Even signs of irritation or frustration may signal his desire to talk. He may use eye contact or a touch to reach out to you. Rely on your intimate familiarity with your partner to sense when he is ready to talk, but waiting for you to make the first move.

Keep the communication going.

Initial conversations may reveal unexpected emotions in your partner. He may even direct his anger and frustration toward you. Don't let that prevent you from sharing your concerns with him in the future. It may be unpleasant at times, but it is necessary. Remind yourself that his negative feelings are really caused by the cancer, not by you.

Through the ups and downs of cancer therapy, open communication may lapse and resentments may fester. The emotional realities between the two of you may hinder openness. This can happen in any marriage, regardless of the circumstances. But this is not a time to stop talking with each other. Communication won't bring an easy resolution to the problems you and your husband face, but it will allow you to face those problems together.

In the war on prostate cancer, the weapons are wielded by physicians. The scalpels, the linear accelerators, the radioactive seeds, the pills, the injections: these are the weapons of destruction in this war. When the cancer is destroyed, the war is won. But the fact that you're not on the front lines of the battle shouldn't minimize your role in winning this war. You represent the home front. You work to keep morale high. At times you may have feelings of helplessness. But your support role is a vital one, and there are many things you can do to help your husband win this war.

Create a comforting environment on the home front.

For most men, home is their refuge from troubles. But cancer brings trouble into the home. Changed roles and family upheaval may turn his household into a stressful environment.

Make every effort to keep the lines of communication open so that an atmosphere of mistrust does not develop. When necessary, work with your husband to reorganize family responsibilities so as to make the transitional period as smooth as possible. Your spouse may feel despondent if he has been suddenly thrust into a state of dependence. While remaining sensitive to his feelings, focus on immediate problems in a pragmatic way. Let him know these changes are just temporary and for the sake of expedience.

Try to keep everyday life on an even keel by maintaining your family's regular routine. A sense of the familiar at home will help compensate for the chaos that has entered your husband's life.

Learn with your partner

Show interest in your husband and his problem by joining him in learning about prostate cancer, its implications and treatment. What you learn will help you understand better what your husband is up against. At the same time, you can encourage your husband to become better informed.

After I told Nancy about my prostate cancer, she took me by the hand and we headed over to the local bookstore. This started me on the way toward taking charge of what was happening to me. Education is a great antidote for the sense of helplessness cancer can create, in both you and your spouse. As in my case, gathering information may reveal a solution to your partner's problem that he did not know existed.

Support his treatment decisions

Along with learning more about prostate cancer at home, you can accompany your husband when he has an appointment see his doctor. Don't insist if he doesn't want you to come. However, in many cases, he will appreciate the support.

Although you may feel pushy, be sure to ask questions about anything of concern to you. The doctor may not know what is important to you, or may feel uncomfortable revealing certain information until asked. And because physicians tend to be busy people, they may not even realize that they have left out certain details. Questions about treatments and their side effects, medications, nutrition, physical and emotional problems all are appropriate areas of concern. Writing questions down before seeing the doctor is a good idea. Be sensitive to your husband's feelings if he is present during your questioning. You may want to talk to the doctor separately about certain issues. If you do, avoid hiding information from your husband that he has a right to know.

Feel free to talk with your partner about various treatments and their possible complications. Let him know your concerns. However, when it comes time to choose a medical treatment, you may have to leave the final decision to him. It is his body, and ultimately his life.

This may be very difficult at times. Nancy felt strongly that the radical prostatectomy was the best way to go. She was concerned about the relatively new nature of the treatment that I chose at the time. Although she found this frustrating, she ultimately supported my decision.

If you feel very strongly that your spouse is making a poor decision, and constructive discussion has not changed his mind, further dispute is unlikely to do any good. If you believe it might sway his decision, you could ask him to talk with a professional, a physician or counselor who could advise him. If this should fail, let him know that even though you disagree with his choice, you respect his right to choose. Then stand by him.

Keep him involved in life

Your partner is almost certain to experience some degree of isolation. The impact of cancer on his life may cause him to withdraw. He may not be physically able to do some of the things he did before. His work or usual activities may no longer be available outlets for him. And because so many people find it uncomfortable to be around someone with cancer, he may sense the outside world withdrawing from him.

Because you are closest to him, make an effort to act as a connection between him and the outside world. At times you may be so busy that you find yourself leading a separate life from him. If so, try to arrange your schedule in order to spend time together and involve him in your life. Stay in contact with friends and relatives, and urge them to call or visit. Encourage your husband to remain as active as he can, without pushing him to doing anything he truly doesn't feel up to doing. He may need some responsible pursuits to keep life purposeful. And without fun and recreation, life becomes dreary.

Pain, fatigue and depression may be interfering with your husband's ability to remain active. See what you can do to mitigate these debilitating influences. Join him in finding creative alternatives to the things that are now missing from his life. With a little effort, you can find positive ways for your partner to stay involved.

Help him to help himself

Many prostate cancer patients are encouraged to make lifestyle and dietary changes to improve their health and fitness. You can be a vital aid in any self-help program he chooses to undertake. Design a menu that provides good nutrition and takes advantage of our current knowledge about the health-promoting powers of certain foods. Naturally, you shouldn't deny him the occasional indulgence in foods he enjoys, or force him to eat what he doesn't like. Even smoking shouldn't be denied him if he wants to continue. If he does not want to quit, encourage him to cut back.

Remember that these changes in his lifestyle are made because they have been statistically shown to provide an advantage in cancer prevention and treatment. Even so, they alone cannot determine whether he will recover from prostate cancer or not. In fact, robbing him of his pleasures may only serve to lower his spirits, which might counteract any good that would otherwise result from healthy lifestyle changes.

Your loving support can also help your husband fight off the emotional effects of prostate cancer. This doesn't mean you always have to be up and energetic around him. Sometimes, commiserating with him over your struggles together will let him know someone shares in his suffering. Talk with him often so you can better understand how he is feeling, and how you can help. Rather than giving him false hope, try to find ways to inspire his realistic hopes. Your positive attitude can work to revitalize his own sense of optimism.

Reassure him of his manhood

Many of the consequences of prostate cancer and its treatments can undermine your husband's feelings of masculinity. He may also no longer be able to assume the traditional male role in the family. Loss of energy and changes in physical appearance can make him seem less robust. Certain drugs used to treat prostate cancer may also make him appear less manly, particularly to himself. The most profound change of all may be his loss of sexual desire or ability, a relatively common complication of the various therapies for prostate cancer.

As a result of his condition, your husband's sense of manhood may be at an all-time low. Like many wives, you may be most concerned about the physical welfare of your husband. Consequently, you may not fully appreciate the terrible pain this attack on his virility is causing your mate.

There are several things you can do to help avert the profound loss of self-esteem that may result. Let him know that your love for him is not a consequence of his physical characteristics but of his personal qualities, which remain unchanged. And though his body image might have suffered, even little things like getting his help opening a jar or bringing in the groceries may bolster his sense of masculinity. Most of all, physical contact will indicate your continued affection for him. Try to tell your partner through touch or word that physical closeness with him remains important to you. Hugging, cuddling and caressing will reassure your husband that you find him desirable, and will be a comfort to you as well.

Showing affection for your husband may sound simple, but sometimes can be very difficult, especially if you are feeling less desirable because he is no longer approaching you. But physical withdrawal from each other will only make it more difficult to restore closeness later on. Again, finding a support group with others that share these problems may be a great help to both of you.

Give him your love

Love is the greatest gift you can give to your husband. There is a reason we always hear about the magical quality that love possesses: because it is true. I know from my own experience that the power of love to heal and restore is immeasurable.

Love is also undoubtedly the fundamental reason for your desire to help your husband or partner. While you are offering your support, take the time to remind him why. Reminders of your love can ease his burden and reassure him that life is worth living. In this way, you can do for him what no one else can. Of all the things you do on his behalf, put loving him at the top of your list.

Overcoming The Threat To Intimacy

For most men with prostate cancer, aside from the threat to life itself, the threat to sexual intimacy is their greatest concern. Fortunately, there is no reason to assume that treatment for prostate cancer will end a man's sex life. However, it is true that the disease and complications of treatment can affect a man's sexual relations. More than a little ingenuity and adaptability may be needed to overcome sexual difficulties should they develop. It is a sad fact that some men and their partners surrender unnecessarily in the face of these difficulties. Some couples give up an active sexual relationship, and some even withdraw from physical closeness altogether. But there are measures that couples can take to keep safeguard their intimacy.

Changes in appearance and sexual capabilities can be frightening. Many of these fears are intensified by the sexual myths that men first encounter in their adolescent years. Such myths may include: A real man never fails to achieve erection. A real man is always ready and willing. A real man is rugged, strong and vigorous. As baseless as assertions may be, when faced with a sexual problem, many men are misguided and troubled by these ingrained notions of masculinity.

It is in the interest of every man to see through these myths, whether he is struggling with a sexual problem or not. For all of us, age undermines those physical attributes that our youth-oriented culture identifies with sexuality. But the process of aging is also an opportunity to more fully appreciate the deeper personal qualities that enrich our intimate relationships. As the importance of the physical aspects wane, the emphasis that we give to mental, emotional, and spiritual aspects of sexuality often grows. This isn't to say that aging and physical changes have no significance. But don't overestimate them. If you feel less attractive, remember that your wife married a person, not a body. Your body may have changed, but you are still the same person you always were.

Similarly, complications of treatment may be troublesome, but they need not end your sex life. Hygienic precautions may be necessary, but no degree of incontinence need bar a man from engaging in sexual activity. Men who suffer problems with erectile function after surgery or radiation therapy still experience desire and can still feel all the sensations associated with sex, including orgasm. Although the situation may be difficult to adjust to emotionally, erectile problems are essentially mechanical in nature and do not really reflect on your manhood. There are many remedies for erectile dysfunction (see Chapter Twelve: Coping with Side Effects). Don't let embarrassment or fear of rejection keep you from seeking a workable solution.

Men who are receiving hormonal therapy may suffer a significant loss of desire as well as erectile dysfunction. This is because in some mysterious way, male hormones are intimately involved in sexual arousal. However, a minority of men undergoing this type of therapy remain sexually active and continue to feel desire. In a way, these men prove the axiom that the brain is the most important sex organ. Although the urge may have diminished, more men might be capable of remaining sexually active if they learned how to encourage the more subtle sexual feelings that the mind can create.

After any form of treatment for prostate cancer, reinitiating sexual involvement with your partner may involve some element of risk, especially when a sexual problem exists. In overcoming any feelings of inadequacy you may have, it may help to better understand your partner's feelings about the matter. Many men have misconceptions about their spouse's sexual needs and desires, and this is where listening to your partner can be a great virtue.

These issues of intimacy are often a topic of discussion during meetings of Side by Side, a support group sponsored by Man to Man for the wives of prostate cancer patients. It is not uncommon to hear a woman testify, "I've loved my husband all my life. We've had a wonderful sexual relationship. I know what he's gone through, and I'm very content with being loved, having a lot of attention, having a special friend, hugging, kissing, and cuddling. We're doing more of that now, and I feel better than I did when we were able to have sexual intercourse." Such testimony underscores the importance of physical closeness and affection as an integral part of a woman's needs.

Before sexual expression can be reintroduced into your marriage, you will need to talk openly with your partner. Communicating about this sensitive subject can be uncomfortable for us, but it is really the only way to come to terms with the issue. Prolonging silence on the subject will most likely lead to a growing distance between you and your partner. And because many women are not sexual initiators, they usually find it at least as hard as their husbands to broach the subject. Your wife may also be avoiding the issue of sex for fear of making you feel inadequate. Let her know you miss being intimate with her and would like to talk about ways of restoring your sex life.

Most therapists suggest gradually reintroducing sexual intimacy into your relationship after treatment. You might want to intentionally limit sexual expression to physical closeness and cuddling at first to alleviate feelings of anxiety. Try to keep the atmosphere light and undemanding. This will enable both you and your partner to more easily come to terms with possible changes in your sexual relationship.

If you are simply unable to openly communicate with your partner about sex, or if you cannot overcome negative thoughts and feelings associated with a sexual problem, it may be appropriate to see a therapist or counselor, that is, a healthcare professional who is trained in treating sexual problems. This type of therapy may involve discussion and "homework" assignments for the couple aimed at establishing better communication, reducing anxiety, and learning new sexual skills. The American Cancer Society provides booklets for men and women who wish to rekindle sexual expression after cancer treatment.

Keeping your sex life going can be a challenge in face of the obstacles that prostate cancer and its treatment often pose. Things may never be the same as they were before. Sex may not be spontaneous. Intercourse may be less frequent. Yet making the effort to restore your sexual relationship with your partner can give you the opportunity to find new means of intimate expression. Some couples may find that their physical relationship has been hindered by treatment side effects, but many of these couples discover a deeper emotional intimacy in their marriage by striving to remain close. In a healthy relationship, there will always be ways of showing love and affection for each other. This is something that can never be taken from you.

CHAPTER ELEVEN

THE FINANCIAL SIDE OF PROSTATE CANCER

I f you have been recently diagnosed with prostate cancer, dealing with the expense of your medical treatment may be far down on your list of concerns. In fact, your immediate reaction may well be, "Forget about the cost! Just help me!" It's true that the financial burden is usually not the worst part of having this disease. But the cost of care is indeed one of the associated pains of prostate cancer. And the sooner you deal with the financial issues involved, the better off you will be.

While it is crucially important for patients to become informed about their treatment options, it also pays to become informed about the financial alternatives to cover medical care. While you are looking after your physical well-being, look after the health of your bank account as well. How? Take a close look at your personal finances to assess the burden that medical treatment might impose on you. Take the time to learn about cost-cutting benefits that may be available to you. Find out how to get the most out of your insurance and/or Medicare coverage. Take steps to prepare yourself for the medical bills that will eventually begin to pile up. Acting early will save you much anxiety later on.

The Cost Of Prostate Cancer Treatments

According to a nationwide UCLA study published by the American Cancer Society in 2000, the average costs for surgery and radiation were as follows:

RP (alone)	$19,019
EBRT (alone)	$15,937

Seeds (alone)	$15,301
RP with Adjuvant EBRT	$31,329
EBRT with Seeds	$24,407

The more technologically advanced forms of external radiation (IMRT, Conformal Radiation, Protons and Neutrons) tend to be more expensive than conventional EBRT. At my institution, the cost of a course of IMRT can be $35,000 or more, not including hospital fees and lab tests. Estimated cost ranges of some of the other common forms of therapy are as follows:

Cryosurgery	$15,000–$18,000
Orchiectomy	$2,000–$3,500
Lupron®, annually	$5,000–$7,000
Zoladex®, annually	$4,000–$6,000
Eulexin®, annually	$2,000–$4,000

According to the UCLA study cited above, "The mean charges for the workup, treatment, and 6 month follow-up of patients treated for early stage prostate carcinoma ranged between $15,301 and $31,329," with significant differences according to the type of treatment *(Cancer 2000 Oct 15;89(8):1792-1799)*. According to a more recent study examining the costs of treating those patients with advanced disease, the average total cost of hospitalization, tests, physician fees, palliative procedures and hormonal therapy was $24,660 over the course of the last year of treatment *(Prostate Cancer Prostatic Dis. 2002;5(2):164-6)*.

Counting The Costs

Medical treatment for cancer doesn't come cheap. This is no less true of the treatments for prostate cancer. The figures cited above provide a general dollar range for the most common forms of therapy for prostate cancer. Note that these prices reflect what a patient would pay if he was personally liable for the full cost of treatment. The actual fees physicians and hospitals receive for a particular treatment differ depending on the source for payment. Medicare, Medicaid, HMOs, and large employer group plans often pay agreed-upon reduced rates for medical services. Furthermore, the price of a particular procedure may vary considerably from doctor to doctor and hospital to hospital. The estimated costs of primary treatment listed above do not include the costs associated with treating complications following primary therapy.

Health Insurance: Avoiding A Financial Fall

Most Americans have some form of health insurance to help cover medical expenses. Given the high costs of medical care, health insurance is often our only protection against financial disaster. Ideally, like a parachute, your insurance plan should save you from potential catastrophe, break your fall, and set you down safe and financially secure. But don't presume that your insurance coverage will necessarily cover all the bills. Your actual liability can vary considerably depending on the type of insurance you possess. Before you take the plunge and get medical treatment, take the time to review your coverage. Some plans have holes you need to watch out for. You need to fully understand how your insurance works. Otherwise, you might just end up in free fall.

The first thing for you to do is get out your insurance policy and carefully examine its provisions and limitations. You will probably see some kind of deductible which must be paid before coverage kicks in. A coinsurance payment is also common. This is the percentage of all claims that you will have to pay, usually ranging from 10% to 25% of those for which you are eligible. Most plans also set a maximum limit to coverage for treatment of a particular condition.

Carefully note the exclusions in your policy. Some of the things that insurance policies may refuse to cover include experimental therapies, home-care services, prosthetic devices, and cosmetic surgery. Preexisting conditions are also usually excluded from coverage. If you are not covered by the policy, or if you do not have insurance, you may still be eligible for some kind of financial assistance.

Types Of Insurance Plans: What Color Is Your Parachute?

Along with knowing the conditions of your policy before medical treatment, it's also important to understand the type of plan under which you are insured. As you are probably aware, in recent decades, the health insurance industry has gone through a revolution. Efforts to control the rising costs of medical care have spawned new breeds of health insurance. There is now a dizzying array of insurance alternatives available to the consumer. At the same time, an already complicated field has become all the more confusing to the average individual. Along with the traditional indemnity plans, there are the plethora of managed-care plans, such as HMOs, PPOs, IPAs, EPOs, and others.

What effect will the type of plan you possess have on your treatment alternatives or quality of care? What should you watch out for with a particular plan? How can you avoid mistakes that might cost you money? Take a brief look at the general types of coverage described below.

The Indemnity Plan

There are basically two types of traditional health insurance plans: indemnity plans and service plans. An indemnity plan pays out a fixed amount of dollars, reimbursing the policyholder for all eligible medical services. For example, a fixed amount is set for each day of hospitalization, usually between $100 and $300. The payment is made directly to you. If you are insured under an indemnity plan, you have the significant advantage of being able to select your own physician. The flexibility of such a plan enables you to take a greater role in assuring that you receive quality care.

There are some drawbacks to indemnity plans. They are usually not very comprehensive in the coverage they provide. Furthermore, you must file claims to receive reimbursement from the insurance company. You will be responsible for all medical costs not covered by the plan. This can sometimes lead to unpleasant surprises. Insurance companies issuing this kind of policy establish a fee schedule, which indicates what the insurer considers the "reasonable and customary" charge for a particular service.

The reasonable and customary fee schedule can vary from company to company. When a large company like General Motors or Microsoft provides medical benefits to their employees, the company may not want to administer the plan. Instead, the plan is farmed out to the administration to another company. That second company may be one like Blue Cross/Blue Shield that will exact a fee for administrative services, but doesn't collect any premiums from covered employees. The original company, GM or Microsoft, is the one that deducts the premium from employees' paychecks. Then, the company will pay Blue Cross/Blue Shield their fee, at the same time maintaining a fund from which employee claims are paid.

What is a reasonable and customary fee? Whatever a company like GM or Microsoft is willing to pay, which is why fees vary. Most employees are unaware of whether or not their employer is self-insured in this manner and are encouraged to believe that the insurance company decides what to pay.

Based on region, the insurer sets a line, usually between 80% and 90% of what physicians typically charge within a community. If your physician charges more than the insurer's set fee, you may be charged with the remainder of the bill on top of your deductible and coinsurance payment. This is a practice known as "balance billing," and the bill can be quite high. For example, urologists in Florida may charge anywhere from $5,000 to $7,500 as their surgical fee to perform a radical prostatectomy. Your insurance company might set $5,500 as the "reasonable" rate for the procedure. If your preference runs toward pricey physicians, you may end up with an unexpected bill from your doctor for $2,000 or more.

There are precautions you can take to avoid or at least reduce such unexpected costs. Check with your doctor to find out how much he charges for a procedure. If you don't feel comfortable asking the doctor directly, talk with your physician's office manager. Also ask for the appropriate "CPT" code or codes for the treatment. Insurers use these codes to identify a medical procedure for reimbursement. Contact your insurance agent, or call the customer hotline provided in your policy, and find out if they will cover the entire fee. If not, see if your physician is willing to perform the procedure "under assignment." This indicates that the physician agrees to accept the insurer's reimbursement fee as payment in full. Also check to see that any hospital or medical facility involved in your treatment accepts assignment.

If you cannot get a procedure done under assignment, you may want to check around for a less expensive center for treatment. However, even if you do end up being treated and "balance billed" for medical services, you may still reduce the bill by negotiating with your physician. Doctors aren't in the business of alienating their patients. Usually, an equitable settlement can be reached.

The following are additional tips if you have indemnity coverage:

Keep careful records.

Copy and keep track of all of your medical bills: Each time you send in a claim, make a copy of the claim form and any attached medical bills and doctor's statement. Also keep records of the reimbursement you receive.

Submit a claim for all medical expenses.

There is no penalty for sending in a claim for bills not covered by your policy. And you never know when you might receive payment for something you did not expect.

Appeal any rejected claim you believe is mistaken.

If you believe your insurance company has unfairly refused to reimburse you, or has not given full reimbursement for treatment, you have the right to appeal their decision. See Fighting For Your Rights later in this chapter for a discussion of the appeal process and other actions you can take to protect your rights.

The Service Plan

Under a service plan, the insurance company arranges with physicians and hospitals to pay a pre-established fee for each medical service. Under plans such as a Blue Cross and Blue Shield service plan, you need only demonstrate to the hospital or physician that you are a member and they will bill the insurance company on your behalf. The insurer pays the provider directly. If you go to a doctor or hospital that has a contractual relationship with the insurance carrier, you will not need to worry about any additional charges beyond your deductible and coinsurance payment. Service plans are usually more comprehensive than indemnity plans.

On the down side, you may be restricted to providers who are "members" of the service plan to receive coverage. Always check to see if your doctor or hospital is a currently participating member of your service plan. Call your insurance agent or your insurer's customer hotline for verification of membership. Your insurance company will provide you with a list of participating providers if you wish to find alternative providers in your area. The doctor's billing department can also verify participation.

In some cases, the service plan allows you to go to non-member doctors and medical facilities. In such an instance, you run the risk of being "balance billed" for any amount beyond what the insurer considers "reasonable and customary" fees for the medical services provided. If your doctor or hospital is not a member of the plan, take the precautions previously detailed under The Indemnity Plan to minimize your liability.

Managed Care

Managed care is now the dominant trend in the health care industry. There are many variants of managed care, but all seek to reduce the costs of medical treatment while providing more comprehensive coverage to plan members. These plans seek to keep costs down by removing the incentives for performing unnecessary tests and treatments.

Different types of managed care companies utilize different strategies to achieve the same end. Health maintenance organizations, or HMOs, often hire their own doctors and may own their own medical facilities. Physicians under contract with an HMO usually receive a salary or a set monthly fee, with the understanding that they will provide any needed medical services to the HMO's enrollees. Independent practice associations, or IPAs, contract with local physicians and hospitals to provide care for their enrolled membership. Unlike most HMOs, IPAs usually reimburse medical service providers on a fee-for-service basis. Preferred provider organizations, or PPOs, also contract with community providers. Physicians and hospitals are guaranteed a volume of patients, with the condition that they accept significantly discounted fees off their posted "sticker prices."

Managed care programs are more comprehensive in their coverage than traditional plans. Premiums are usually about the same as a traditional plan, but deductibles and coinsurance payments, if any, are nominal. Out-of-pocket expenses are generally kept to a minimum. Periodically, you will receive an "explanation of benefits" (EOB) detailing all the services the managed care provider has paid on your behalf.

The benefits of a managed care plans are offset by certain disadvantages. These plans are often very restrictive, and limit their subscribers to a select list of physicians and hospitals. You may find that none of the physicians you have access to have significant experience performing a given procedure or a particular treatment option may not even be available to you!

Under some managed care plans, you may go outside the designated list of providers, but only at a considerable penalty. PPOs and point-of-service plans typically offer to pay 70% for doctors outside the plan's network, although this is based on a fee schedule that the insurer considers "reasonable and customary." If your physician is expensive, you may end up paying far more than 30% of the bill.

The pressure within managed care plans to reduce unnecessary medical services sometimes results in a tendency to undertreat medical problems. Physicians and hospitals may suffer economically if they treat certain conditions aggressively. Patients with expensive diseases such as cancer are those most likely to suffer due to the stress on cost-cutting in managed care organizations.

With managed care plans, decisions regarding your care are made by your primary physician, called the "gatekeeper" physician. Before you can receive coverage for a diagnostic test, treatment or hospitalization, your doctor must receive pre-approval from the insurance company. The insurer may deny authorization for any medical service deemed to be non-standard or experimental. Because a managed care company must reduce costs to remain profitable, the pressures to deny care can be considerable. Again, see Fighting For Your Rights to find out what to do if you believe you have been unfairly denied care.

Financial Aid

Perhaps your insurance coverage is inadequate. Even worse, you may not have any insurance at all. Once diagnosed with cancer, it can be virtually impossible to obtain insurance coverage for your condition. If you're lucky, you may have access to a group plan that does not screen for pre-existing conditions. In addition, during open enrollment periods, Medicare HMOs must accept everyone who is eligible, regardless of medical conditions. Still, in many cases the only insurance you may be able to buy will contain a provision to exclude a pre-existing condition such as prostate cancer. Fortunately, there are government programs that may help reduce your medical expenses. Following is a discussion of financial aid alternatives you may be eligible to receive.

Medicare

Medicare is a federal program originally designed to provide health care to the elderly. Those age 65 or older are eligible to apply for coverage. Because prostate cancer is a disease that afflicts men in their later years, a large percentage of men with prostate cancer qualify for Medicare coverage. Disabled individuals are also eligible.

Medicare is divided into two parts: Part A, hospital insurance, and Part B, supplemental medical insurance. When you enroll for Social Security benefits, you are automatically covered under Medicare Part A, which covers hospitalization, in-patient nursing care, home health care, and hospice services. There is a large annual deductible, which was $840 for the year of 2003. Part B is voluntary and requires payment of a monthly premium. Part B is more comprehensive, covering such things as doctor's fees and some outpatient services. It has a lower deductible and requires a 20% coinsurance payment. Medicare pays for some medical services, but certainly will not cover all your medical costs. Many individuals with Medicare choose to purchase supplemental insurance to cover costs Medicare does not.

Medicare is essentially an indemnity insurance program. Claims must be filed, and Medicare reimburses the patient for all eligible medical services received. The processing of claims is not performed by the government directly. Instead, private companies serve as intermediaries to handle claims and make payments. These intermediaries determine what services are covered and how much to reimburse. After a claim is processed, you will receive an "explanation of Medicare benefits" (EOMB) in the mail describing what Medicare paid, how much was credited to your deductible, and what claim charges were rejected.

It's important to make sure any hospitals or physicians whose services you intend to use are Medicare certified. Medicare usually will not reimburse providers who lack Medicare certification. If you are covered by Medicare Part B, make sure that your physician uses Medicare certified laboratories as well. Also note that under current policy guidelines, Medicare does not reimburse prostate cancer patients for medications taken orally (such as Eulexin®), but does cover those drugs taken by injection (such as Lupron® and Zoladex®). It should also be noted that many drug companies offer discounted prices through "compassionate programs" for Medicare eligible patients.

Medicare reimbursement rates are often considerably less than the going rate for a medical service. Check to see if your doctor or hospital will provide services to you "under assignment." If so, they explicitly agree to accept Medicare's reimbursement for all eligible medical services as payment in full. Any provider of medical services that is a "Medicare participating provider" cannot charge the patient more than the Medicare-allowed rate for a Medicare-covered service. Participating providers are also required to file claims directly on your behalf. When services are not provided under assignment, you are responsible for fees in excess of the Medicare-allowable reimbursement rates. However, you may still be able to negotiate a reduced rate. Under current law the patient is responsible to pay 20% of "Medicare allowable," which cannot be discounted unless the patient can demonstrate a "financial hardship." In many cases, supplemental insurance may cover the difference.

It is essential that you follow proper procedures in filing claims. Your Social Security office will give you free assistance in completing claim forms. Keep in mind that Medicare will only cover services determined to be medically "reasonable and necessary." Application of this provision is often difficult and subjective. You may have to rely on your physician to define services that Medicare will reimburse. You do have the right to appeal rejected claims if you feel that reimbursement has not been justifiably denied. More on the appeals process may be found under Fighting For Your Rights.

The federal Medicare program is also experimenting with managed care. Those patients who enrolled in Medicare Part A and Part B are eligible to enroll in a Medicare-contracted HMO, if one is operating in their area. Medicare HMOs provide more comprehensive coverage than traditional Medicare, often for the same monthly fee, but require you to see only their doctors.

Medicaid

Medicaid is a program operated by individual states under federal guidelines to provide financial aid for those with limited resources. The benefits and conditions of Medicaid vary considerably from state to state. Federal guidelines require certain minimum services be provided to individuals on Medicaid. Individuals who are disabled or receive federal or state aid are usually eligible for Medicaid. To apply, contact the state or local department of social services. Information on your income and assets is required to determine eligibility for Medicaid.

Other Alternatives

There are still other alternatives for financial aid. Disability insurance is available to anyone who is unable to work due to a serious and long-term disability. To find out if you are eligible, contact your local Social Security office. Veterans who lack funds to pay for their own medical care can take advantage of their benefits offered through the Veterans Administration. The VA has hundreds of specially designated hospitals across the country. Several states also sell comprehensive health insurance for residents who cannot find a company to insure them due to a serious medical condition. Contact the state department of insurance to find out if there is such a program in your state. Entering a clinical trial may be an option for reducing costs, as most expenses are paid for by the sponsor of the trial.

Finally, many city and county governments also have programs to provide medical services for local residents. Those who are not covered by private insurance, Medicare or Medicaid can take advantage of these programs. Contact the social service agencies of your local government, or the county health department, to find out what programs are available to those who are at a disadvantage in paying for medical care.

Fighting For Your Rights

In a perfect world, no problems with your health insurance would ever arise. But in reality, such conflicts are commonplace. Regardless of the specific type of health insurance you have, you may find yourself in a dispute with your insurer.

Perhaps you believe that a claim has been unfairly denied. Perhaps the insurer has refused to cover a particular form of therapy. There are certainly examples of this in the case of prostate cancer, especially with therapies still considered investigational, which may not yet be accepted by insurance carriers. Even traditionally accepted therapies can sometimes run into problems. One HMO effectively denied coverage for external radiation therapy by requiring pre-approval for each of the 30 or so treatments!

If you find yourself in such a situation, you have rights as a consumer that you can exercise. And according to surveys, more than half of the individuals who contest a denial of benefits win their case against the insurer. But one thing is for sure: no one else will defend your rights for you. You have to take the initiative to fight for your rights.

What To Do If Coverage Is Denied

You may be denied insurance coverage before or after receiving treatment. In many prepaid plans, pre-approval for treatment may be refused, indicating that the insurer will not cover your costs if you proceed with treatment. With indemnity plans or Medicare, a claim you submitted may be denied following treatment.

In contesting a denial of coverage, it is very important to follow proper procedure. Health plans use different grievance and appeal processes. If you are denied coverage, look in your "evidence of benefits" brochure to find out about the specific grievance or appeal procedures available in your plan. You may wish to contact the consumer representative at the plan's member services office should you desire help filing a formal complaint.

The following are tips that may help you as you fight for your rights:

Utilize your rights under Medicare.

If you are covered by Medicare, by law the hospital or physician must provide you with written "notice of non-coverage" if it is believed Medicare will not cover a particular service. This notice contains an explanation as to why Medicare will not pay. You may feel the medical provider's notice of non-coverage is mistaken, in which case you have the right to order a claim be submitted to Medicare on your behalf anyway. Your claim will then be reviewed by a Peer Review Organization (PRO), a group of doctors who are paid by the federal government to oversee treatment through Medicare. The PRO may review and reject your claim, in which case you may request reconsideration of your claim by the PRO at a later date.

Check for clerical errors.

When a claim is rejected or not paid in full, it may be the result of a simple clerical error. You should have copies of the claim form and medical bills to compare with the notification of denial. If you find the problem is some simple mistake, a phone call or letter can usually resolve the dispute.

Look at the reason given for denying coverage.

The reason may be that the insurer has deemed the treatment is not a "medical necessity," or is "nonstandard" or "experimental." Definitions of these terms vary from plan to plan. Before responding, check the definitions in your policy. You will need to provide evidence or a second opinion to show the reason given for denial is wrong.

Ask for your doctor's help.

When you request reconsideration from the insurer or Medicare intermediary, your physician can best explain why a particular treatment is not experimental in nature, and why it was medically necessary in your case. Your doctor may also be able to help when you are simply seeking full reimbursement of a claim. Insurers will often increase reimbursement beyond the customary fee if there is an explanation of extenuating circumstances. Additional documentation is essential if you are to get your insurer to overturn their previous decision in your case.

Medicare recipients may request reconsideration on decisions by their peer review organization.

If the determination to reject your claim came from the regional peer review organization that oversees Medicare reimbursement, your first step in appealing is to request a reconsideration. Contact the PRO and ask for the specific procedures you should follow in making an appeal.

Make it clear that you mean business.

When making a written request for reconsideration to your insurance company or Medicare intermediary, structure your request as a formal business letter. Be sure to include your policy and claim numbers. Let them know that you are giving them the opportunity to reevaluate their denial of coverage. Indicate that you are currently preparing to appeal this denial and wish the insurer to provide you with additional written documentation. Also indicate that consecutive copies are being sent to all concerned parties, such as your physician or your group plan administrator. If you have a lawyer, be sure to include his or her name (for example, "cc: John Smith, Esq."). Be persistent. If within two or three weeks there is no response or notice of payment, send your written request again, with SECOND NOTICE printed at the top.

If necessary, take matters farther.

If your claim continues to be denied, you may choose to pursue the matter further. If your claim was denied by a PRO or Medicare intermediary, you may request a hearing by an administrative law judge. If a considerable amount of money is involved, you can eventually appeal to a federal court. Many private insurance plans require binding arbitration for quality-of-care and denial-of-benefits disputes. Arbitration avoids legal costs to the insurer, but you may have to pay arbitration fees. Note that these appeal mechanisms may involve considerable time and expense, and should only be undertaken after other avenues of reaching a resolution have been unsuccessful.

Hire a lawyer.

If serving as your own advocate does not solve the dispute, hire an attorney to work for you. Resorting to a lawsuit can be effective. Try to find a lawyer experienced in insurance claims. Under legal pressure, insurance companies will often pay for new forms of therapy otherwise labeled as "experimental." If an insurance company thinks it will cost more to deny coverage, threat of a lawsuit may induce the company to pay up.

File an insurance complaint when treated unfairly.

Insurance regulators are another resource you have at your disposal. They possess the power to conduct investigations, hold hearings, impose fines, and compel reimbursement of offended parties. You should be ready to follow through on your complaint if necessary. This may involve responding to additional requests for information and appearing at hearings. If you have a good case, however, the end result may be a resolution of the dispute in your favor.

Contact the government agency that regulates your insurer to inquire about the proper procedure for filing a complaint. If your insurer is a private company, contact your state department of insurance and the state's insurance commissioner. Those who are insured by Medicare or belong to a federally qualified health maintenance organization (such as a Medicare HMO) should file complaints with the U.S. Health Care Financing Administration or U.S. Social Security Administration. Insurance plans administered by a large employer are regulated by the U.S. Department of Labor.

Your Health Is Worth The Price

The rising cost of health care is an important problem. But most people find ways to pay for the care they need. However, sometimes that means making tough choices. You may find that the treatment you choose is influenced by monetary concerns. Is there any price that is too high when it comes to your health? Only you can make that decision for yourself. But first take every step to minimize your financial strain. If you do, you may never have to face this question. And you'll also be able to stay focused on the most important thing—winning your battle against prostate cancer!

PART THREE

BY JENNIFER CASH, ARNP, MS, OCN®

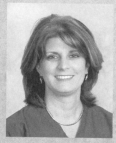

In my capacity as an Advanced Registered Nurse Practitioner (ARNP), I am often the first care provider to have contact with patients prior to treatment. We nurses, as frontline caregivers, are in a unique position to guide patients with support and reassurance throughout their course of treatment and recovery. Through education about the disease process, the treatment procedure and its associated side effects, we strive to deliver a high quality of care with a holistic approach that takes into account the physical, emotional and mental health of our patients.

POST-TREATMENT CARE AND LIFESTYLE CHANGES

As a member of a brachytherapy and radiation oncology team, I routinely counsel patients as well as their families before, during and after treatment. In the pages that follow, part of my discussion of side effects and quality of life concerns is directed to those patients undergoing radiation therapy. This group of patients now represents the majority of those being treated for localized prostate cancer. However, many of the specific comments and guidelines offered here also apply to surgical patients and others who may experience treatment-related side effects such as erectile dysfunction or incontinence.

CHAPTER TWELVE

COPING WITH
SIDE EFFECTS

As Dr. Dattoli indicated in his discussion, all of the primary, curative treatments for prostate cancer carry some risk of temporary and long-term side effects. Even men who are successfully treated may find their triumph over the disease eclipsed by the subsequent complications of their treatment. The most common and distressing complications are incontinence and erectile dysfunction. Fortunately, there are a variety of therapies available to help patients cope with these untoward side effects. In addition, there are a number of remedies to reduce or ameliorate the short term side effects commonly experienced by men who undergo brachytherapy and external radiation therapy.

Post-implant Side Effects

While brachytherapy carries the lowest risk of permanent complications, most seed implant patients experience short term side effects such as urinary obstruction or urethral irritation, which may include frequency, urgency, decreased flow of the urine stream, difficult or painful discharge of urine (dysuria) and getting up at night to urinate (nocturia). Rectal symptoms are uncommon; however, some patients do experience soft stools and/or increased frequency of bowel movements. Perineal discomfort immediately following treatment is usually minimal and easily remedied by oral steroidal and non-steroidal anti-inflammatory agents and mild analgesics. Sitz baths (sitting in warm water for 15 to 20 minutes) or ice packs may also be used to treat rectal or perineal discomfort. Some patients may also experience painful ejaculations that resolve with time.

The duration of urinary and rectal side effects is shorter with palladium implants than with iodine implants because of palladium's shorter half-life. Immediate postoperative urinary side effects may occur 7 to 10 days after the brachytherapy procedure. With Pd-103, symptoms usually peak in severity within 2 to 4 weeks, but they may persist at a higher level for 2 to 3 months. With I-125, these same symptoms may last 10 to 12 months. There are many factors that may influence the duration of urinary symptoms, including prostatitis, enlarged prostates, dietary intake, and non-compliance with prescribed medications. These are routinely managed as indicated. *It should be also noted that patients who have received IMRT prior to brachytherapy, do not experience any significant increase in the temporary side effects associated with implantation.*

At our institution, after a patient is discharged following brachytherapy, a number of medications are commonly prescribed. These include the following:

➤ An anti-inflammatory to help reduce swelling of the prostate. Typically, a steroid anti-inflammatory will be used for several days, and thereafter a non-steroidal anti-inflammatory such as ibuprofen.

➤ An over-the-counter medication like Pepcid AC may be used with the anti-inflammatory to prevent stomach upset.

➤ An antibiotic is routinely prescribed to prevent infection of the prostate.

➤ An alpha-blocker such as Flomax®, Uroxatral®, Hytrin® or Cardura® is prescribed to aid the flow of urination. This is the most important medication for the treatment of urinary symptoms. Patients usually continue using an alpha-blocker for several weeks to several months, depending on the duration of symptoms.

➤ Hydrocortisone suppositories are used as a preventative medication to ameliorate any rectal irritation that may result from the ultrasound rectal probe used during the seeding procedure, or from irritation caused by the radiation, or from pre-existing hemorrhoids.

➤ Over-the-counter medications such as Azo Standard or Azo Cranberry, sodium bicarbonate tablets, or Prelief® may be used to help with any urinary burning or discomfort.

➤ Over-the-counter preparations such as Metamucil or Citracel may be used for constipation or looseness of the bowels.

It should also be noted that radiation patients are advised to avoid all antioxidant supplements such as Vitamins A, C, E, beta carotene and selenium, as these may have an opposing action to the radiation treatment (see Chapter Thirteen: Diet and Nutrition Guidelines).

Common Bladder Irritants Post-Seeding

After brachytherapy, the following foods may cause painful or more frequent urination. Some men can tolerate limited amounts of these foods, while other men cannot. 6 to 8 weeks after seeding, patients can try to slowly reintroduce these foods into their diets. Keep in mind this is not an exhaustive list, and patients may find they are sensitive to other foods as well.

- Apricots
- Alcoholic beverages
- Apples
- Avocados
- Bananas
- Beer
- Brewers Yeast
- Caffeine
- Cantaloupes
- Carbonated drinks
- Champagne
- Cheese (aged)
- Chicken Livers
- Chillies
- Chocolate
- Citrus Fruits / Juices
  (especially with fortified Vitamin C)
- Coffee (even decaf)
- Corn Syrup
- Fava Beans
- Grapes
- Lemon Juice
- Lima Beans
- Milk Products
- Mayonnaise
- Nuts (in general)
- Nutrasweet
- Onions
- Peaches
- Pineapple
- Plums
- Foods High In Potassium
- Rye Bread

- Saccharine
- Sour Cream
- Soy Sauce
- Spicy Foods
- Strawberries
- Tea
- Tomatoes
- Vinegar
- Vitamins Buffered with Aspirin
- Yogurt
- Sugar
- Honey

Milder Substitutes

The following milder foods can be substituted for those on the previous list of common bladder irritants. These items should be used sparingly and on a limited basis for the first 6 to 8 weeks after treatment. Remember, each individual is different, so these foods should be introduced slowly into the patient's diet in order to gauge his reaction.

- Alcohol or wine for flavoring
- Almonds
- Apple – small
- Blueberries
- Cashews
- Carob
- Coffee – acid free
- Kava or highly roasted
- Extracts (Rum, Brandy, etc.)
- Fish
- French Sauternes
- Frozen Yogurt
- Garlic
- Imitation Sour Cream
- Melons
- Onions – cooked
- Peanuts
- Pears
- Pine Nuts
- Poultry
- Processed Cheeses (not aged)
- Shallots
- Spring Water
- White Chocolate
- Zest of Oranges or Limes

Urinary Incontinence

Urinary incontinence (involuntary urine leakage or dribbling) is a common side effect after radical surgery, however, it also affects a very small percentage of men treated with radiation. Incontinence may be temporary or in some cases permanent. It is also influenced by previous surgeries of the bowel, bladder and prostate (TURP). The severity of the condition varies widely, from mild stress incontinence to overflow or urgency incontinence, which is the inability to delay urination when the bladder feels full. Depending on the cause and severity of the incontinence, a number of effective treatments are available.

Incontinence is more than a physical disorder. If left untreated or managed improperly, it can affect quality of life. If you are a patient having difficulty with urinary control, you may feel embarrassed about discussing the problem, but keep in mind that you are not alone and there are effective remedies. You may harbor feelings of anxiety or anger, or you may feel isolated because of the condition. Fear of having an accident may prevent you from taking part in normal activities. By reporting the problem to your doctor, he can evaluate the nature and extent of the condition and recommend an appropriate treatment option or options. These may include one or more of the following:

Medications

If only partial damage has been sustained by the muscles controlling retention of urine, various drugs such as Ephedrine® can be used to contract the remaining muscle tissue. This treatment can restore or improve continence in many cases. Other drugs such as Detrol®, Ditropan® and Oxytrol™ may also be used to relax the bladder and reduce the pressure it exerts on stored urine, thereby minimizing leakage.

Kegel exercises

Special exercises are another technique often used to treat incontinence. Kegel exercises involve alternate tightening and relaxing of the sphincter muscles at the base of the pelvis, as if trying to hold in urine. These exercises can help restore lost urinary control for many men. A study in 2003 at the Kaiser Permanente Medical Center in Los Angeles found that surgical patients who did Kegel exercises regained control of continence faster than men who didn't exercise. Biofeedback may also be used to train and strengthen the muscles that control urination.

Collagen Injections

Collagen is an insoluble protein found in the connective tissues of the joints and bones. Purified into a white, fibrous paste, collagen is injected into the neck of the bladder to narrow the urethral opening. Men whose urethral sphincter has been damaged by surgery may be good candidates for this treatment. The procedure used to inject the collagen takes about 30 minutes and is relatively inexpensive.

Artificial Sphincters

If drug therapy and physical therapy are unsuccessful and the patient is not a good candidate for collagen injections, then surgery may be used to treat incontinence as well. An artificial sphincter may be implanted to control urine flow. An inflatable cuff is placed around the urethra, usually just below the external urethral sphincter. Once inflated, the flow of urine is cut off. When the need to void is felt, a pump mechanism can be triggered that will deflate the cuff and allow urine to flow out of the bladder. Even in the most severe cases of incontinence, these artificial sphincters can often dramatically improve the condition.

Even in cases where the incontinence cannot be completely corrected, there are a number of ways to manage the problem and enable men to carry on a normal lifestyle. Developing a regular schedule for drinking and voiding can reduce many problems associated with incontinence. With men who are overweight, shedding some pounds can significantly improve urinary control by reducing pressure on the bladder. Avoidance of diuretic foods and drugs will also promote continence. There are also numerous absorbent products and devices that are comfortable and allow men to remain active, regardless of the degree of incontinence. These range from absorbent pads and drip collectors to adult briefs and undergarments. Bed pads and absorbent mattress covers can also be used to protect the mattress and bedding.

Although incontinence can be an unpleasant problem to deal with at times, through care and planning, the possibility of embarrassment can be avoided altogether. With the wide range of treatments and products now available, any man can learn to go about his life without having to withdraw from society and without giving up any of the activities that he enjoys.

Erectile Dysfunction (ED)

Erectile dysfunction is a possible outcome of any form of treatment for prostate cancer, although there is a higher risk with radical surgery and cryosurgery than with seed implants and IMRT. Even patients who undergo nerve-sparing prostatectomies may experience impaired sexual function. ED is also a common side effect in men who have had orchiectomies and those who are prescribed hormonal agents.

Men who are in their later years and no longer sexually active are not likely to be concerned about this complication. But most patients who are still sexually active before treatment will be anxious to take some action to restore any loss of ability to achieve an erection. There is no simple test for erectile dysfunction. The only way for a doctor to know that a sexual problem exists is through statements from the patient himself. To complicate matters, sexual problems may have both psychological and physical causes. Sometimes merely anticipating erectile problems after treatment will cause men to experience a loss of normal erectile function. Stress, anxiety and depression can also contribute to the problem. More recently, smoking has been found to be a profound contributor to erectile dysfunction, as are obesity and diabetes.

A diagnostic analysis is usually the first step in treating potency problems. This entails detailed questioning to ascertain the nature of the problem. If the ability to achieve an erection varies depending on the time or circumstances, then at least part of the problem is likely to be psychological and may be treated through counseling. To determine if there is a physical basis for the problem, a doctor may perform tests to measure blood pressure and pulse in the penis. These may indicate that circulation problems are impairing the patient's ability to have an erection. A blood test may also be used to check the level of male hormones. Because many men experience erections during sleep, a sleep laboratory evaluation is sometimes performed. Normal erections experienced during sleep indicate that the problem does not have a physical basis.

In many cases, however, a physical cause for erectile dysfunction will be found. There are several potential physical causes of these side effects. Both surgery and radiation can damage the nerves or proximal penile tissue that control erection. Vascular damage may be another cause of sexual dysfunction after treatment, as damage to the blood vessels can reduce the blood flow to the penis needed to achieve an erection. Certain medications, such as those used to treat high blood pressure and depression, may also contribute to erectile problems.

A number of treatment options are available for men suffering from erectile dysfunction. These include the following:

Phosphodiesterase inhibitors. Drugs such as sildenafil (Viagra®), vardenafil (Levitra®), and tadalafil (Cialis®) have been very effective in helping to restore erectile function after treatment. With brachytherapy and IMRT, more than 90% of men who were sexually active prior to treatment are able to retain sexual function post-implant. With surgical patients, Viagra® is significantly less effective and will not work for men who have had both neurovascular bundles removed or damaged. According to one study, erectile function was preserved in 71% of patients undergoing bilateral nerve-sparing RP, 50% of patients undergoing unilateral RP, and 15% of those men who had RPs without utilizing the nerve-sparing procedure (Zippe CD et al, Urology 55: 241-245. 2000).

Viagra® and similar drugs increase blood flow to the penis to help achieve and maintain a satisfactory erection. These drugs only work when a man is sexually stimulated, and do not increase sexual desire (libido). They can cause side effects including headaches, flushing, indigestion, light sensitivity and other visual problems, and runny or stuffy nose. Most of these side effects are mild and short-lived, however, in some cases more serious problems can occur. Patients who experience prolonged erections (four hours or more) should seek medical attention immediately.

Interactions with other drugs are also possible, so be sure your doctor knows what medications you are taking. Drugs that contain nitrates, which are often used for treating heart disease, can interact with these potency drugs to cause very low blood pressure, a potentially fatal complication. The use of Viagra®, Levitra® and Cialis® may also be contra-indicated for patients who are taking alpha blockers (Flomax®, Hytrin®, Cardura®, Minipress®, Uroxatral®), as the interaction with these medications may cause a similar drop in blood pressure. Before taking any of these potency drugs, you should inform your doctor if you have a history of heart problems, low or high blood pressure, a history of stroke, kidney or liver problems, stomach ulcer, blood cell abnormalities, Peyronie's disease, or any other significant health problem.

Injections. A variety of other drugs can be used to treat erectile dysfunction. Papaverine, Phentolamine, and Prostaglandin E1 are drugs used to relax muscles and increase the blood supplied to the penis. Injections are made directly into the penis, initially by the physician and later by the patient himself. Although many men find the idea of penile injections unpleasant, they cause only minimal discomfort.

Men uncomfortable with needles can get a simple device that automatically injects medication with the press of a button. Prostaglandin E1 can also be applied to the surface of the penis or inserted in the form of a urethral pellet (Muse®), thereby eliminating the need for injections. For many men, these medications have proven very effective in restoring lost erectile function, but for those who have had extensive damage to the blood vessels in the vicinity of the prostate, due to surgery, cryosurgery or radiation therapy, these drugs may be ineffectual.

Penile Implants. Intrapenile prosthetic devices can be a satisfactory solution for men who wish to continue having intercourse. A penile prosthesis is surgically inserted inside the shaft of the penis. The penile implants currently available fall into two basic categories: those that are inflatable and those that are semi-rigid. The advantages and disadvantages of each type of prosthesis should be discussed by the patient and his physician. Men should also include their partners in decisions about implants and other erectile aids.

Vacuum Devices. These non-surgical devices use vacuum suction and penile constriction to assist blood flow into the penis, causing an erection. They consist of a plastic cylinder placed over the penis and a hand-held pump to draw air from the cylinder. Once an erection is achieved, an elastic band is placed around the base of the penis to maintain erection. Although less popular than injections or implant devices, these devices are often effective and have the advantage of being non-invasive.

Surgical Treatment. For those patients who suffer from vascular blockage that does not respond to other treatments, an experimental surgical procedure may be performed. An artery that usually supplies blood to the stomach is rerouted by the surgeon and connected to blood vessels inside the penis. Results with this procedure so far have been not been very successful.

Over the Counter Products. There are also over the counter products to improve sexual perfomance. Supplements that may help include zinc, L-Arginine, Yohimbe, Chrysin, Avena Sativa, stinging nettles, Tribulus, and Muira Pauma. It should be noted that testosterone enhancers, replacements and boosts may be contra-indicated for men with prostate cancer due possible increased risk of recurrence.

These various treatments enable many men with erectile dysfunction to enjoy normal sexual relations. However, one should be realistic about what these methods can and cannot do. Those who suffer from low sexual desire or decreased sensation may not be entirely satisfied with the results that these treatments provide.

Beyond the various treatments for erectile dysfunction, certain changes can be made to counteract other factors that may be contributing to the sexual impairment. Medications that contribute to an erectile problem or a loss of sexual desire can often be exchanged for others that do not have these side effects. Other complications, such as pain or fatigue, may also be contributing factors. Treating these conditions may help. Lifestyle changes, such as improved diet, exercise, quitting smoking, and reduced consumption of alcohol, can also lead to improved sexual performance. When psychological or emotional issues are involved, counseling may serve to decrease performance anxiety and overcome mental blocks to satisfying sex.

CHAPTER THIRTEEN

DIETandNUTRITION GUIDELINES

Diet and Prostate Cancer

There is a growing body of evidence that indicates there is a close connection between diet and prostate cancer, as well as other forms of cancer. Other than genetic make-up, no factor has greater influence on a man's likelihood of developing prostate cancer in later life than his diet. We know there is a link between diets high in saturated and total fat and an *increased* risk of prostate cancer. On the other hand, we also know there is a *decreased* risk of prostate cancer with men whose diets are high in fiber, phytoestrogen ("phyto" is Greek for plant), lycopenes (another phyto chemical) and other nutrients.

Recent studies also indicate that dietary habits may improve the prognosis of men already diagnosed with prostate cancer, regardless of stage. It's never too late to change unhealthy eating habits, and it makes good sense for prostate cancer patients to improve their chances for recovery by adopting a healthier diet. If you are undergoing treatment for the disease, your first priority should be to maintain your strength and overall health. In this regard, diet will play an important role before, during and after the treatment process

General Dietary Guidelines

There is no definitive diet for preventing or treating prostate cancer. Specific changes in diet depend on the individual patient. At our institution, we advise patients to consult with a physician or qualified nutritionist for help in developing an individualized diet plan. It should be noted that there is no evidence that diet alone can cure prostate cancer, and therefore, no one should attempt to use diet or nutritional supplements as substitutes for medical treatment. However, in general, there are a number of steps that men with prostate cancer can and should take to enhance their prospects for overcoming the disease.

Eat A Low-Fat Diet

Many studies have implicated excessive fat consumption with the development of cancer. The average American man gets approximately 35% or more of his total calories from fat in his diet. The American Cancer Society recommends reducing total fat intake to no more than 30% of total calories for all men and women, including cancer patients. Limiting dietary fat in this way may be especially important in retarding the development of prostate cancer.

A number of studies have demonstrated the link between prostate cancer and a high-fat diet. We know that the incidence of prostate cancer is highest in countries where high-fat diets are prevalent. Prostate cancer is considerably less common among Asian men than men in the U.S., yet the rate of incidence for Asian-Americans who have adopted a typical American diet closely approaches that of other Americans. Studies also show a connection between fat in the diet and mortality rates from prostate cancer. A study from the Harvard School of Public Health found that men with prostate cancer who ate high-fat diets had a 79% greater chance of developing advanced disease. This risk increased significantly when the fat came from red meat.

Given what we know, the most effective way to reduce your risk is to cut down on animal fat in your diet. Favor lean meat and don't eat red meat more than once a week. Instead, you might eat white fish and skinless poultry. Limit your consumption of dairy products. Avoid saturated fats and heavy oils, such as butter, margarine, shortening and corn oil. Instead, polyunsaturated oils, such as olive or safflower oils, should be used in cooking. In addition, avoid heavily processed foods, fast foods and snack foods, all of which are usually high in fat.

The percentage of body fat, not just fats consumed in foods, is also a factor contributing to the growth of prostate cancer. According to the

American Cancer Society, overweight people have roughly twice the cancer mortality rate of people who aren't overweight. Obesity also complicates surgery for prostate cancer, may contribute to symptoms of the disease, and increases the likelihood of heart disease and other health problems. All in all, men with prostate cancer who are significantly overweight would do well to reduce their level of body fat. For patients with an obesity problem, the best course may be a physician-assisted weight loss program, which may also utilize the American Dietetic Soup Diet, Weight Watchers, or similar programs.

If you have prostate cancer and you are one of the millions of Americans who are currently on one of the popular low-carb diets (i.e. the Atkins diet, South Beach diet, the Zone diet), you should consider modifying the plan with your doctor to conform to American Cancer Society recommendations for patients with prostate cancer. The ACS guidelines are similar to those of the American Heart Association and the American Dietetic Association. There is general agreement among nutritionists that a healthy diet involves reducing fat intake and placing more emphasis on fruits and vegetables. The ACS suggests 5 or more servings of fruits and vegetables each day. Grain products, bread, cereals, rice, pasta, and beans are also recommended.

Reduce Cholesterol To Healthy Levels

The media often characterizes cholesterol as a potentially deadly substance, but in reality most cholesterol is manufactured by the body itself for the building of cellular membranes and the formation of vital hormones. The dangers associated with cholesterol occur when supply exceeds demand. Excess cholesterol has been strongly linked to heart attacks and strokes, and may contribute to erectile problems in some men. Although the evidence is so far inconclusive, some researchers suspect high cholesterol may also play a role in prostate cancer.

An overall cholesterol level that exceeds 240 milligrams per deciliter (mg/dl) may signal a problem. But the component elements of blood cholesterol are also relevant. Cholesterol comes in two forms: low-density lipoproteins (LDLs) and high-density lipoproteins. Research shows that low levels of high-density lipoproteins (HDLs) may pose as great a health risk as high total cholesterol levels. It appears that higher than average levels of HDL cholesterol can reduce the odds of future health problems. In general, it is wise for men with prostate cancer to reduce their cholesterol levels to around 180 to 200 mg/dl, while maintaining HDL levels at about 45 mg/dl or higher.

Common sense might suggest that the best way to reduce your cholesterol level would be to eat foods low in cholesterol. But dietary cholesterol actually has little impact on blood cholesterol. However, there is a close correlation between dietary fat and the level of serum (blood) cholesterol. Once again, saturated fats are the major offender. Reducing fat intake is the most effective means to lower cholesterol through diet. Substitution of monounsaturated fats for saturated fats will help to lower LDL levels while maintaining the level of HDL's in your bloodstream.

Other dietary changes also have an impact on cholesterol levels. There is evidence that added fiber in the diet can significantly lower cholesterol. Patients are well advised to limit dietary cholesterol from meat and dairy sources to 300 mg/day or less. This is about as much cholesterol as found in 12 ounces of ground beef, 6 ounces of steamed shrimp, or 1 ½ eggs.

Another important factor in managing cholesterol is exercise, which can boost HDL levels by as much as 10% to 20%. In contrast, smoking can significantly reduce HDL levels. When all else fails, certain drugs can effectively treat high cholesterol. Your physician will be able to advise you on whether drug treatment would be appropriate in your case.

Maintain A Varied Diet

Most dietary experts recommend a varied diet of nutritious foods. This used to mean that a daily diet should include portions from the four basic food groups: meat, dairy, grains, and fruits and vegetables. The four food groups have since been supplanted by the food pyramid in the U.S. Department of Agriculture's updated dietary guidelines. Breads, cereals, pasta and grains serve as the foundation—three to six servings each day, including several whole grain products. Five to ten servings of fruits and vegetables each day are recommended. Meat, poultry, fish, and other protein sources should be limited to two servings each day. Recommended daily consumption of dairy sources is likewise two servings per day in a healthy diet.

The guidelines are based on research that shows the foundation of a healthy diet to be whole grains, fruits and vegetables. On the other hand, the role of the meat and dairy groups, once seen as staples of a nutritious diet, are significantly diminished. Current USDA recommendations suggest a diet high in fiber, low in fat, and rich in complex carbohydrates. The USDA also strongly advises limiting the consumption of fats, sweets, and alcoholic beverages.

Those contemplating or currently practicing vegetarianism should not interpret the reduced significance of meat and dairy in the new dietary recommendations as sufficient reason for eliminating these food groups entirely. Without proper care, a vegetarian diet may supply inadequate levels of essential amino acids, and could lead to nutritional deficiencies, such as a deficiency of zinc, a mineral central to prostate function. However, with proper planning, a varied vegetarian diet can supply all the essential nutrients.

This underscores the importance of practicing variety within food groups as well. A diet in which vegetable content is supplied only by corn and potatoes will be deficient in many essential nutrients. The relatively recent discovery of phytochemicals, naturally produced chemicals in plants that possess an apparent ability to block carcinogenic processes, indicates that the well-established vitamins and minerals are not the only compounds found in plants that provide health benefits. Frequent rotation of foods, especially whole foods, is one way to ensure a varied, nutritious diet.

Eat Cancer-Fighting Foods

While a healthy diet ought to provide all the nutrients needed by the body, research indicates that certain vitamins, minerals, and chemicals found in foods are particularly useful in combating cancer. These natural substances use a number of mechanisms to protect the body from cancer formation and proliferation. The following may be of use in the fight against prostate cancer:

Vitamin D

Some epidemiological studies, which track broad patterns of diet and disease in the population, suggest that vitamin D may help prevent prostate cancer. In fact, several studies indicate that exposure to sunlight can significantly reduce the risk of prostate cancer, possibly due to the skin's conversion of sunlight into vitamin D. Besides sunlight, the best sources for this vitamin are sardines, fortified milk, and egg yolks.

Antioxidants

This group of nutrients include vitamins A, C, E, selenium and beta-carotene. They are all the rage these days in the popular media and with health-conscious consumers, as evidence is slowly accumulating that these substances may provide protection against cancer, heart disease, and other disorders.

According to current theory, antioxidants work to block the formation in the body of dangerous forms of oxygen known as free radicals. These free radicals are believed to damage cell membranes, impairing the cell's ability to perform essential tasks, such as control of metabolism, regeneration of internal damage, and elimination of bacteria, viruses and toxins. If this theory is correct, antioxidants may help to short circuit the processes that lead to cancer. Studies thus far have been inconclusive, but including foods in your diet that are rich in antioxidants may be beneficial.

Overcooking food can eliminate these important nutrients, and because many vitamins are water-soluble, they can be lost through boiling. Therefore, it is best to eat fruits and vegetables raw or steamed. Those patients concerned that their diet is not supplying sufficient quantities of these important nutrients can supplement their diet with a multivitamin. Further supplementation should be undertaken only under a doctor's supervision. In addition, as previously noted, patients undergoing radiation therapy should avoid excessive antioxidants while being treated, as these may have an opposing action to radiation. For more information on specific antioxidants, see Nutritional Supplements below.

Phytochemicals

These substances are naturally occurring chemicals found in plants, apparently serving to protect them from the harmful effects of sunlight. Medical research has shown that phytochemicals also serve as cancer-fighting agents in the human body. A myriad of these biochemicals exist in the fruits and vegetables that we eat—it's been estimated that there are 10,000 in tomatoes alone! Although they have yet to draw the media interest generated by the antioxidants, phytochemicals have caught the attention of private and public institutions in the health industry. The National Cancer Institute has launched a multimillion-dollar project to isolate and study them.

There is some evidence indicating the microscopic activities of these chemicals may slow or reverse the mechanisms that lead to the growth of malignant tumors. Para-coumaric acid and chlorogenic acid, found in tomatoes as well as several other fruits and vegetables, block the formation of carcinogenic compounds called nitrosomes. A phytochemical in turnips eliminates enzymes that cause cellular mutations. Sulforaphane, one of many phytochemicals found in broccoli, has been shown to retard the development of breast tumors in mice.

According to researchers, phytochemicals work by synthesizing enzymes that attach to carcinogenic molecules, dragging them out of the cells before any damage can be done. Citrus fruits, berries, and a number of vegetables contain flavanoids, phytochemicals that prevent cancer-causing hormones from fastening onto cells. These chemicals might be especially advantageous to prostate cancer patients, since most cases of prostate cancer are hormone-dependent.

Another significant finding for men with prostate cancer is a chemical in soybeans called *genistein,* discovered by German researchers. Genistein acts to prevent the formation of capillaries around a malignant tumor, essentially cutting off the tumor's supply lines to impede or halt its growth. This finding has prompted some researchers to suggest that one cause for the high risk of prostate cancer among Asian men who emigrate to the U.S. may be due to the adoption of a soy-poor American diet.

Although synthetic versions of sulforaphane have been created in the laboratory, in all likelihood it will be many years before phytochemicals will be available in a pill. Until then, make sure you eat plenty of whole fruits and vegetables. Fortunately, most phytochemicals appear to hold up through a variety of cooking processes.

Zinc

The prostate gland contains higher concentrations of zinc than any other part of the body. The exact relationship between zinc and the prostate is unknown, but there is some evidence suggesting that a zinc deficiency may precede the development of prostate problems, including prostate cancer. For this reason, eating foods containing zinc may be beneficial. Foods rich in zinc include pumpkin seeds, oysters and other seafood, nuts, wheat bran and wheat germ, milk, eggs, onions, poultry, gelatin, beans, peas, lentils, and beef liver. Overcooking will deplete the natural zinc content of most foods.

Zinc supplements are sometimes prescribed to treat the symptoms of prostate enlargement and prostatitis, and should only be taken under the supervision of a physician. It should also be noted that there is not yet any solid evidence that zinc supplements are effective in treating prostate cancer.

Nutritional Supplements

Vitamins are natural substances that have been scientifically established to be essential for physical health. A deficiency in any of the essential vitamins may result in serious health problems, such as scurvy or rickets (due to deficiencies of vitamins C and D respectively). The development of natural and synthetic vitamin supplements was aimed at the prevention of such deficiencies. Now most deficiencies can be prevented or corrected through the use of nutritional supplements. Taking vitamin or mineral supplements may affect your prostate cancer risk, but this is not yet clear.

The therapeutic value of vitamin and mineral supplements such as antioxidants—vitamins A, C, E, beta-carotene and selenium—is still the subject of debate. When it comes to the health benefits of nutritional supplements in excess of the recommended daily allowances (RDAs), the opinions of physicians and other health professionals vary to some degree. Many conventional physicians question the value of using vitamin megadoses (recommending higher doses than the RDA) as a form of therapy, arguing that megadosing is an expensive and potentially hazardous health fad, driven primarily by profit.

Proponents of the medicinal use of vitamin and mineral megadosing argue that even though scientific proof is inconclusive, the public should not be denied information on potentially beneficial alternatives. No doubt the debate will continue. There are a number of specific antioxidants that may be beneficial for men with prostate cancer, and these are discussed below.

Vitamin A (retinol) and Beta-carotene

In its active form, vitamin A is found only in animal products such as whole milk, eggs, and meat, especially liver. Because many of these foods should be eaten in moderation, it is probably better to rely on the vitamin A precursor, beta-carotene, for this valuable nutrient. Found in a wide range of fruits and vegetables, beta-carotene is essentially two vitamin A molecules linked together. The liver acts to convert beta-carotene into active vitamin A.

Both animal studies and human trials have demonstrated a connection between low levels of these nutrients in the diet and increased risk of a variety of cancers. However, some studies have suggested that vitamin A supplements may actually *increase* the risk of prostate cancer by lowering the level of zinc in the prostate. The evidence to date points to beta-carotene as a better antioxidant and more effective anticancer agent.

When taken at high doses for a prolonged period, vitamin A can cause harmful, even fatal, liver damage. Dietary supplementation with beta-carotene is a much safer approach. Excessive dosages (megadosing) of beta-carotene may cause a yellowing of the skin (carotenosis), but this condition appears to be harmless.

Vitamin C (ascorbic acid)

Nobel Laureate Dr. Linus Pauling, who popularized the use of vitamin C as a remedy for the common cold, also advocated the use of vitamin C supplements for the prevention and treatment of cancer. Vitamin C is not only a powerful antioxidant, but plays an important role in the immune system. During the 1970s, Pauling published several studies that showed high doses of supplemental vitamin C increased survival time for terminal cancer patients. However, at least three randomized trials by the National Cancer Institute failed to confirm Dr. Pauling's findings, and subsequent studies have been inconclusive.

Orange juice, as well as tomatoes, broccoli, Brussels sprouts, cabbage, green peppers, and spinach, are good sources of vitamin C. The RDA for vitamin C is 60 milligrams, but the vitamin is generally considered nontoxic at much higher dosages. The most common side effect of excessive vitamin C is diarrhea. Rare complications have been known to result as a consequence of megadosing. Also, the body becomes conditioned to higher intake of vitamin C, and abrupt cessation of a high dosage could result in a dangerous drop of vitamin C in the blood. Dosages far in excess of nutritional needs should only be taken in consultation with a physician.

Vitamin E

This antioxidant vitamin has been the subject of much attention. Foods rich in vitamin E include green leafy vegetables, whole grains, and vegetable oils. Like vitamin A, vitamin E is a fat-soluble vitamin that's collects in the body. However, vitamin E appears to be safer than vitamin A in large doses. Still, researchers caution that the safety of vitamin E megadoses taken over an extended period has not yet been established.

Some studies suggest that taking 50 milligrams (or 400 International Units) of vitamin E daily can lower risk for prostate cancer. Although other studies found vitamin E to be of no benefit, reasonable doses of this vitamin have no significant side effects and are not expensive. Vitamin E works synergistically with selenium in the body, and taking them in conjunction may enhance their beneficial properties.

Selenium

Found in meat, seafood and whole grains, selenium is an essential trace mineral needed by the body for pancreatic function and to maintain tissue elasticity. Selenium is also a broad-spectrum antioxidant. Studies have shown that selenium and vitamin E work together to aid in the production of antibodies. Animal studies have found selenium retards tumor formation. Other studies suggest that ending selenium supplementation in animals can result in an increase in tumor development. Therefore, those who advocate taking selenium to prevent cancer also caution against sudden cessation of supplementation.

As with vitamins A, C, and E, several studies have found that individuals with low serum selenium levels had a significantly higher risk of developing cancer. A large-scale NCI study—the Selenium and Vitamin E Cancer Prevention Trial (SELECT)—is currently underway to investigate the effects of selenium and vitamin E supplementation. Unfortunately, the results of this study will probably not be available until 2013.

The RDA for selenium is 70 micrograms, but it has been argued that only megadose quantities on the order of several hundred or more micrograms can successfully increase blood levels of selenium. Some patients have difficulty absorbing selenium when taken as oral supplements. Caution should be practiced in taking large doses of selenium, since the mineral can be quite toxic. Bad breath is one harmless side effect of selenium megadoses, but more severe symptoms can result as a consequence of selenium toxicity. These include nausea and weakness. There may also be discoloration of the fingernails. Close medical supervision and testing of blood selenium levels is necessary to prevent toxicity in those taking large doses of selenium.

Additional Suggestions

The patient is the one who must finally decide whether or not to take nutritional supplements. The safest route—and one recommended by the FDA—is to get your antioxidants in the foods you eat every day. Nevertheless, you may wish to take more aggressive action. If a blood test indicates that you have low levels of key nutrients in your bloodstream, you may be more likely to benefit from supplements. But keep in mind that megadosages can be hazardous, and some supplements may interact with various medications or pose a health risk for men with medical conditions other than prostate cancer. Always seek the advice of a physician before beginning any vitamin regimen.

Although much has been made of studies indicating the promise of antioxidants as cancer-fighting agents, nutritional supplements are no substitute for a proper diet and healthy lifestyle. Don't make them a substitute for practicing healthy habits in your life. In addition, it should be noted again that supplements may help to prevent prostate cancer, but after cancer is diagnosed, they will not bring about a cure. All prostate cancer patients require appropriate medical treatment to be cured or to minimize progression of the disease.

Summary of Diet and Nutrition Guidelines

At the Dattoli Cancer Center, patients who are being treated for prostate cancer are routinely advised as follows, with appropriate updates as new studies continually improve our current knowledge:

In general, eat healthy with a higher protein, lower fat diet

Adopt a mainly vegan diet consisting of fruits and vegetables (5 servings a day), and legumes. Minimize or eliminate red meat entirely. Chicken and fish are best if broiled or baked. Fish should be lean (and oily) like Salmon, Tuna, Anchovies, Sardines, Mackerel (which also contains Omega-3 acids). Make sure to remove skin from chicken before cooking. Avoid all fried foods.

Increase fiber intake and limit dairy product consumption

Eat more fruits and vegetables. Eat salads with at least one meal each day, and have two vegetables with dinner. Try going "veggie" for one night a week. Add vegetables to soups and casseroles. Eat fruits for snacks and desserts instead of sweets. Rice, pasta, beans and some nuts (small amount) are good on a daily basis.

Increase Phytoestrogen intake

Concentrate on soybeans and soy products, legumes (beans), bean sprouts, sunflower seeds, rye, wheat and all berries.

Increase Lycopene intake

Increase consumption of tomato-based foods, such as tomato sauce, pizza, and tomatoes.

Increase intake of zinc, selenium and vitamin E

Eat more whole grains and wheat germ.

Avoid fats and oils

Use less butter, margarine, oil and high-fat salad dressings. Use olive oil instead. Consume less cheese, or use fat-free or low-fat cheeses. Eat fewer desserts, or choose low-fat or fat-free desserts.

Decrease alcohol consumption (no more than 1-2 drinks per day) and all caffeinated beverages

Caffeine drinks include coffee, regular tea, and soda.

Incorporate as many of the following in your daily diet as possible:

➢ **Soy products**—soy milk or powder, or genistein.

➢ **Green Tea**—2-3 cups a day.

➤ **Lycopenes**–tomato food sources (juice, sauces, etc.) are preferred but lycopene can be taken in pill form (30mg-45mg daily).

➤ **Vitamin C**–500mg.

➤ **Vitamin E**–400–800 I.U. (a combination of gamma and alpha tocopherol is preferred).

➤ **Calcium Citrate or Carbonate**–400mg at dinner, 400mg at bedtime.

➤ **Saw Palmetto extract**–300mg twice daily (unless taking a "prostate formula" multivitamin supplement).

➤ **Selenium**–200mcg.

➤ **Zinc**–50-100mg.

➤ **Modified Citrus Pectin** (optional).

➤ **CLA (conjugated linoleic acid)**–3 grams (optional).

➤ **Quercetin**–as per instructions (found in health food stores) for general prostate health. You may also use a combination product with Chrysin and Saw Palmetto called Sports One Chrysin XS. Also, Certinin and Indole-3 Carbinol may be used as per instructions.

➤ **Glutamine**–2 grams with each meal and at bedtime (for muscle strength).

➤ **Glucosamine**–1500mg (NOT to be combined with chondroitin).

➤ **CoQ10**–optional because of expense.

➤ **Fish Oil Omega 3 (with or without Rosemary)**–2000 mg 2 times daily.

➤ **Curcumin (from Tumeric)**–200-400 daily.

➤ **Zyflamend**–1 capsule twice daily.

There are a number of prostate antioxidant formulas found in most pharmacies and health food stores, and these may contain the majority of these supplements. They may be easier to take than separate doses of each item above. If you elect to take one of these preparations, make sure it contains folic acid.

Exercise on a regular basis

Without overdoing it, try to exercise at least 30 minutes on most days of the week. Exercise activities might include walking, jogging, swimming, exercise equipment, light weights, etc. At the same time you address diet and fitness, find a form of stress management that works for you. Some type of meditation or yoga for 20 minutes once or twice daily may be helpful for stress relief.

More Diet Guidelines

Another comprehensive source on diet guidelines for prostate cancer patients can be found on-line in the publication, *Eating Your Way to Better Health: The Prostate Forum Nutrition Guide,* compiled by Charles E. Myers, Jr., M.D., et al. For more information, visit the Prostate Forum website at:

www.prostateforum.com/nutrition.htm

The article, "Nutrition for Healing After Prostate Cancer," by Pamela Mathis, M.Ed., R.D., L.D. also offers comprehensive nutritional guidelines for patients and is available upon request from the Dattoli Cancer Center (see *Appendix B: Where To Get Help*).

WHERE TO GET HELP

Your Physician

A trusted physician who is familiar with your case should be your most important source of information and advice. For those who desire additional information, there are a number of organizations devoted to helping prostate cancer patients and their families. These agencies provide information and counseling, and in some cases, they may provide financial aid and/or transportation to a medical facility for treatment.

Organizations and Businesses

The following is a list of national organizations and medical centers that provide information and services for prostate cancer patients. For information on local support groups, contact the social service office of a local hospital, or write or call one of the national cancer information services listed below.

Allegheny General Hospital

Jeffrey K. Cohen M.D.
625 Stanwix St., Suite 1209, Pittsburgh, PA 15222
(412) 281-1757

Allegheny General Hospital is a primary site using cryosurgery for the treatment of prostate cancer. Dr. Cohen has performed many of the cryosurgical procedures done since clinical trials began in July of 1990. Those interested in learning more about this treatment may contact Dr. Cohen at the address or phone number above.

American Cancer Society (ACS)
1599 Clifton Road, N.E. Atlanta, GA 30329
(800) ACS-2345
http://www.cancer.org

Man To Man Prostate Cancer Support Groups
The American Cancer Society is involved in education and research, and offers counseling and other patient services. The Society consists of more than 3000 local chapters across the United States, and has adopted the Man to Man prostate cancer support group program on a national basis.

American Foundation of Urologic Disease
300 West Pratt Street, Suite 401, Baltimore, MD 21201-2463
(800) 242-2383
http://www.afud.org

Amersham Healthcare
Medi-Physics, Inc., 101 Carnegie Center, Princeton, NJ 08540
(800) 654-0118
http://www.amershamhealth-us.com

Medi-Physics is the manufacturer of the radioactive iodine seeds used in brachytherapy for the treatment of early stage prostate cancer. The company readily supplies information to those wanting to know more about seed implantation and Medi-Physics products. Medi-Physics also makes available listings of doctors who perform the seed implantation procedure.

Cancer Information Service (CIS)
National Cancer Institute (NCI) Building 31, Room 10A24 9000
Rockville Pike Bethesda, MD 20892
(800) 4-CANCER
http://cis.nci.nih.gov/

A governmental service that provides information by telephone and via Web site to cancer patients, the public, and health care professionals. Trained staff members can provide information on current treatments, cancer prevention, and the nearest Comprehensive Cancer Center. The

National Cancer Institute also supplies a wide variety of written materials to answer questions about cancer. The PDQ, or Physician Data Query, is a computer information system that provides doctors and patients with the latest information on clinical trials and their results. The Cancer Information Service will provide a copy of the PDQ to anyone who requests it.

Dattoli Cancer Center

2803 Fruitville Road, Sarasota, FL 34237
(877) 328-8654 toll free
http://www.dattoli.com

The Dattoli Cancer Center & Brachytherapy Research Institute specializes in combined treatment modalities that often pairs brachytherapy with Intensity Modulated Radiation Therapy. The authors of this book are affiliated with this facility.

Impotence Institute of America

8201 Corporate Drive, Suite 320, Landover, MD 20715
(800) 669-1603
http://www.impotenceworld.org

Impotence Anonymous

A division of the Impotence World Assocation, the Impotence Institute of America (IIA) is a nonprofit organization dedicated to helping men with impotence problems and their partners. The Institute provides information and physician referrals, and is sponsor of Impotence Anonymous, a support group with chapters in most major metropolitan centers.

Loma Linda Medical Center

Jerry D. Slater M.D.
Proton Treatment Center 11234 Anderson Street
Loma Linda, CA 92354
(909) 824-4288 (800) 496-4966, USA only.
http://www.llu.edu/proton/

Loma Linda University in southern California is the site of the Loma Linda Proton Treatment Center, built in 1991. The Loma Linda center and Massachusetts General Hospital in Cambridge, Massachusetts are currently the only operational hospital facilities that offer proton therapy for the treatment of cancer. Contact the Loma Linda staff for more information on this therapy.

Man To Man

c/o American Cancer Society
1599 Clifton Road, N.E. Atlanta, GA 30329
(800) ACS-2345
http://www.cancer.org/docroot/SHR/content/SHR_2.1_x_Man_to_Man.
asp?sitearea=SHR

Man To Man is a national support group officially sponsored by the American Cancer Society to provide information and support to men with prostate cancer and their families. To find out more about Man To Man, contact the American Cancer Society at the address and phone number listed above.

National Association for Continence

P.O. Box 8306, Spartansburg, SC 29305 (864) 579-7900
http://www.nafc.org

Formerly called Help for Incontinent People (HIP), the National Assoca-tion for Continence is a nonprofit organization that provides information and services to those suffering from incontinence problems.

Patient Advocates for Advanced Cancer Treatments (PAACT)

1143 Parmelee NW, Grand Rapids, MI 49504 (616) 453-1477
http://www.paactusa.org

A nonprofit organization for both patients and physicians that promotes an understanding of prostate cancer, its diagnosis and therapeutic treat-ment. PAACT has a database on thousands with prostate cancer, and read-ily provides information concerning treatment options by telephone and e-mail to those diagnosed with prostate cancer.

Prostate Cancer Research Institute (PCRI)

5777 W. Century Blvd., Suite 885, Los Angeles, CA 90045
Helpline: 310-743-2110
http://www.prostate-cancer.org

The Prostate Cancer Research Institute is a non-profit organization that offers information to patients and physicians.

Schering-Plough Corporation

2000 Galloping Hill Road, Kenilworth, NJ 07033-0530
(908) 298-4000
http://www.schering-plough.com

Schering Corporation is the manufacturer of Eulexin® capsules, a brand name of the anti-androgen drug, flutamide. The company provides a booklet about flutamide and advanced prostate cancer.

Theragenics Corporation

5325 Oakbrook Parkway Norcross, GA 30093
(800) 458-4372
http://www.theragenics.com

Theragenics is the largest manufacturer of the radioactive palladium seeds used in brachytherapy for the treatment of prostate cancer. The company supplies information to those interested in knowing more about the seed implantation procedure and Theragenics' products. Theragenics will also refer interested patients to a physician who offers the seed implantation treatment in their general area.

US TOO Support Groups

US TOO, Inc. 5003 Fairview Avenue, Downers Grove, IL 60515
(630) 795-1002
PCa Support Hotline: (800) 80-US-TOO
http://www.ustoo.com/

The mission of US TOO!™, is to provide counseling, fellowship, and support to cancer patients and their families. Contact the national headquarters of US TOO!™ at the address and number above to find out where your nearest US TOO!™ chapter is located.

Varian Medical Systems, Inc.

1678 S. Pioneer Road, Salt Lake City UT 84104

(800) 432-4422

http://www.varian.com/com

Varian specializes in integrated cancer therapy systems, including Intensity Modulated Radiation Therapy and brachytherapy.

Veterans Affairs (VA) Hospitals and Support Services

The Department of Veterans Affairs (VA) supports veterans seeking the benefits and services earned through military service. For Vietnam veterans, benefits may include disability compensation, health care services, tax breaks, and more. For more information about these programs, call the VA's toll-free Agent Orange Helpline at 1-800-749-8387, or go to the web site at www.vva.org/benefits/vvgagent.htm. The home page for the Department of Veterans affairs is located at http://www.va.gov/. For questions about VA healthcare benefits, call toll free 1-877-222-8387.

Internet Resources

The following is a list of specialized Web sites devoted to prostate cancer information and support:

Prostate Pointers
http://www.prostatepointers.org

Prostate Cancer Profiler
http://www.cancerprofiler.nexcura.com/Interface.asp?CB=66

Prostate cancer acronyms and abbreviations:
http://www.prostatepointers.org/prostate/ed-pip/acronyms.html

Prostate cancer glossary of terms:
http://www.prostatepointers.org/prostate/ed-pip/glossary.html

Prostate Cancer Foundation is the renamed Michael Milken CaP Cure
http://www.prostatecancerfoundation.org/

National Prostate Cancer Coalition:
http://www.pcacoalition.org/

A comprehensive list of PCa papers by Stephen B. Strum, MD:
http://www.prostatepointers.org/strum/

PCa information provided by Charles Myers, MD:
http://www.prostatepointers.org/cmyers

Physician-to-Patient and Patient-to-Patient Web sites:
http://www.prostatepointers.org/p2p

SeedPods (brachytherapy patients):
http://www.prostatepointers.org/SeedPods/

IceBalls (cryosurgery patients):
http://www.prostatepointers.org/iceballs/

List of ED specialists:
http://www.prostatepointers.org/pcai/ed.html

The Circle:
http://www.prostatepointers.org/circle/

Organize your PC digest::
http://www.prostatepointers.org/p2p/pcd.html

Search prostatepointers.org:
http://www.prostatepointers.org/search_form.html

The Education Center for Prostate Cancer Patients:
http://www.ecpcp.org

Prostate Cancer Resource Guide:
http://www.afud.org/pca/pcaindex.html

National Cancer Institute's Prostate Cancer Home Page:
http://www.cancer.gov/cancerinfo/types/prostate

The Hypertext Guide to Prostate Cancer:
http://www.hypertext.org

Florida Cancer Education Network:
http://www.florida-prostate-cancer.org/

Prostate Cancer InfoLink Archive:
http://www.phoenix5.org/Infolink/index.html

PPML website:
http://listserv.acor.org/diseases/prostate

PPML archives:
http://listserv.acor.org/archives/prostate.html

MultiGraph: your medical history in graphic form, free from PC-REF:
Contact John Fistere at JFistere@cox.net
http://members.cox.net/jfistere/MultiGraphIntro.htm

WellnessWeb Prostate Cancer Center:
http://www.wellnessweb.com/PROSTATE/prostate.htm

Center for Prostate Disease Research:
http://www.cpdr.org/

Patients Helping Patients:
http://www.prostate-help.org/

You Are Not Alone:
http://www.yananow.net/

Malecare: lecture transcripts, English and Spanish New York City support
groups:
http://www.malecare.com

Canadian Prostate Cancer Network:
http://www.cpcn.org/

Brotherhood of the Balloon—Proton Therapy Info and Support:
http://www.protonbob.com/homepage.asp

Chemocare.com:
http://www.chemocare.com/splash/splash.sps

PSA Rising Magazine:
http://www.psa-rising.com

Prostate Cancer Action Network:
http://www.prostatepointers.org/pcan/

National Physician & Family Referral Project–PCa in African-American Men:
http://npfr.50hoops.org

Pubmed search–a comprehensive listing of research studies and published papers:
http://www.ncbi.nlm.nih.gov/entrez/query.fcgi

GLOSSARY OF MEDICAL TERMS

3DCRT (3-Dimensional Conformal Radiation Therapy): See Conformal Radiotherapy.

5-alpha reductase (5-AR): an enzyme that converts testosterone to dihydrotestosterone (DHT).

Adenocarcinoma: A cancer originating in glandular tissue. Prostate cancer is classified as adenocarcinoma of the prostate.

Adjuvant: An additional treatment used to increase the effectiveness of the primary therapy. Radiation therapy and hormonal therapy are often used as adjuvant treatments following a radical prostatectomy. Compare Neoadjuvant.

Agonist: A chemical substance that combines with a receptor on a cell and initiates an activity or reaction. See LHRH analogs.

Algorithm: A step-by-step procedure for solving a problem or accomplishing some end, especially by a computer.

Analog: A man-made chemical compound that is structurally similar to one produced naturally by the body. See LHRH analogs.

Androgen: A hormone that produces male characteristics. See testosterone.

Androgen ablation therapy: A therapy designed to inhibit the body's production of testosterones.

Androgen-dependent cells: Prostate cancer cells which are nourished by male hormones and therefore are capable of being destroyed by hormone deprivation (also known as androgen-sensitive cells).

Androgen-independent cells: Prostate cancer cells which are not dependent on male hormones and therefore do not respond to hormonal therapy (also known as androgen-insensitive cells).

Androgens: The male hormones, such as testosterone.

Anesthetic: A drug that produces general or local loss of physical sensations, particularly pain. A "spinal" is the injection of a local anesthetic into the area surrounding the spinal cord.

Aneuploid: Having an abnormal number of chromosomes, as revealed by ploidy analysis. Aneuploid prostate cancer cells tend not to respond well to androgen deprivation therapy (ADT).

Angiogenesis: The body's formation of new blood vessels. Some anti-cancer drugs work by blocking angiogenesis, thus preventing blood from reaching and nourishing a tumor.

Antagonist: A chemical substance in the body that acts to reduce the physiological activity of another chemical substance.

Anti-androgens: Drugs such as flutamide that block the activity of androgens produced by the adrenal glands at the cellular receptor sites. Androgens can block or neutralize the effects of testosterone and DHT on prostate cancer cells (by preventing testosterone and DHT from binding to the androgen receptor).

Antibody: A protein produced by the body that counteracts the toxic effects of a foreign substance, organism, or disease within the body.

Antigen: A foreign substance such as a virus or bacterium that causes an immune response or the formation of an antibody.

Antioxidents: Any substances which delay the process of oxidation in the body.

Apoptosis: The normal molecular mechanism which governs the life span of cells so that they die in a very organized way. Cancerous cells are resistant to normal apoptosis.

Benign: A non-cancerous condition. See also Benign Prostatic Hypertrophy.

Benign Prostatic Hypertrophy (BPH): Also called Benign Prostatic Hyperplasia, BPH is a non-cancerous condition of the prostate that results in a growth of tumorous tissue and increase in the size of the prostate.

Biopsy: A procedure involving the removal of tissue from the body of the patient. Removed tissue is typically examined microscopically by a pathologist in order to make a precise diagnosis of the patient's condition.

Bone scan: An imaging technique used to detect bone metastases, which appear as "hot spots" on the film. It is far more sensitive than the conventional x-ray.

BPH: See Benign Prostatic Hypertrophy.

Brachytherapy: A form of radiation therapy in which radioactive seeds are implanted into the prostate to deliver radiation directly to the tumor. Also referred to as seed implantation, or seeding.

Cancer: A cellular malignancy typically forming tumors. Unlike benign tumors, these tend to invade surrounding tissues and spread to distant sites of the body.

Carcinoma: A malignant tumor made up chiefly of epithelial cells, or those cells that form the lining of an organ or cavity. See Adenocarcinoma.

Castrate Range: The level of the body's testosterone after orchiectomy (also referred to as castration). This is the range or level, which is used by physicians as a point of comparison for those drugs, which attempt to decrease the testosterone level.

CAT Scan (or CT Scan): See Computer Tomography.

cGy: Abbreviation for centigray; a unit of radiation equivalent to the older unit called a "rad."

Chemotherapy: The treatment of cancer using chemicals that deter the growth of cancer cells.

Collimator: A device that organizes radiation such that only parallel rays or beams emanate.

Combination Therapy: A form of hormonal therapy that surgically or chemically blocks the production of testosterone by the testes, and involves the additional use of an antiandrogen to block the receptor sites from utilizing testosterone produced by the adrenal glands. Combination Therapy can also refer more generally to any combination of treatment modalities used to treat prostate cancer.

Computer Tomography: Computer generated cross-sectional images of a portion of the body. Also called CT or CAT scan.

Conformal Radiotherapy: A radiation treatment conforming precisely to the size and shape of the prostate, with the use of computerized planning and state-of-the-art imaging techniques. 3-Dimensional Conformal Radiation Therapy (3DCRT) utilizes this sophisticated approach to treatment planning, as does the even more advanced Intensity Modulation Radiation Therapy (IMRT).

Cryosurgery (also referred to as Cryotherapy or Cryoablation): The freezing of tissue with the use of liquid nitrogen or Argon gas probes. When used to treat prostate cancer, the cryoprobes are guided by transrectal ultrasound.

Cytokine: Any of a class of immunoregulatory substances that are secreted by cells of the immune system.

DHT (dihydrotestosterone): The active form of the male hormone, testosterone, produced after testosterone is transformed by an enzyme known as 5-alpha reductase.

Diagnosis: Evaluation of a patient's symptoms and/or test results, with the intent of identifying and verifying the existence of any underlying disease or abnormal condition.

Digital Rectal Examination (DRE): A procedure in which the physician inserts a gloved, lubricated finger into the rectum to examine the prostate gland for signs of cancer.

DNA (Deoxyribonucleic Acid): A complex protein that is the carrier of genetic information that determines the physical development and growth of living organisms.

Doppler Ultrasound Technique: A machine that sends out ultrasonic waves that pick up the velocity of blood flow through the veins and are transmitted as sound to make an image.

Doubling Time: The time it takes for a tumor or cancerous focus to double in size.

Downsizing: The use of hormonal therapy or other forms of intervention to reduce tumor volume prior to primary, curative treatment.

Downstaging: The use of hormonal therapy or other forms of intervention to lower the clinical stage of prostate cancer prior to primary, curative treatment.

Ejaculatory Ducts: The tubular passages through which semen reaches the prostatic urethra during orgasm.

Ejaculation: The release of semen through the penis during orgasm.

Endorectal MRI: Magnetic resonance imaging of the prostate gland using a probe inserted into the rectum.

Enzyme: A chemical substance produced by living cells that causes chemical reactions to take place while not being changed itself.

Erectile Dysfunction (also referred to as ED or impotence): The loss of ability to produce and/or sustain an erection sufficient for intercourse.

Estrogen: A female sex hormone that can be used as a form of therapy to inhibit the production of testosterone in patients diagnosed with prostate. cancer.

Eulexin®: See flutamide.

External Beam Radiation Therapy (EBRT): A form of radiation therapy that utilizes radiation delivered by an external source (machine) and directed at a target area to be radiated. In contrast to EBRT, brachytherapy utilizes radiation sources (seeds) that are internal, implanted in the target tissue. EBRT may use conventional photons, protons, neutrons or electrons.

Extracapsular Extension: Used to describe prostate cancer that has spread outside the prostate gland.

False Negative: An erroneous negative test result. For example, an imaging test that fails to show the presence of a cancer tumor later found by biopsy to be present in the patient is said to have returned a false negative result.

False Positive: A positive test result that mistakenly identifies a state or condition that does not in fact exist.

Fistula: With regard to prostate cancer, an abnormal passage due to injury or disease that connects an abscess or hollow organ to the surface of the body or to another hollow organ. If there is significant damage to the rectal wall proximate to the bladder, a fistula may occur between the bladder and rectum.

Flare Reaction: A testosterone surge caused by the initial use of an LHRH analog, causing a temporary increase of tumor growth and symptoms (known as clinical flare), or an increase in PSA (biochemical flare).

Flutamide: The generic name of Eulexin®, an anti-androgen used in hormonal therapy for the palliative treatment of advanced prostate cancer and for adjuvant and neoadjuvant treatment of earlier stages of prostate cancer.

Foley Catheter: A catheter inserted in the penis and threaded through the urethra to the bladder where it is held in place with a tiny, inflated balloon. It removes urine from the bladder and can be used to irrigate the urethra and prevent blood clots.

Free PSA: PSA that is unattached to any major protein in the blood. Free PSA is associated with benign prostate growth. The percentage of free PSA is derived by dividing the free-PSA level by the total-PSA x 100. Studies have show that men with free PSA % > 25% were at low risk for prostate cancer, while men with PSA % < 10% were at high risk for having prostate cancer.

Frozen Section: A technique in which removed tissue is frozen, cut into thin slices, and stained for microscopic examination. A pathologist can rapidly complete a frozen section analysis, and for this reason, it is commonly used during surgery to quickly provide the surgeon with vital information.

Gland: An aggregation of cells (a structure or organ) that secretes a substance for use or discharge from the body.

Gland Volume: The size in cubic centimeters (cc) or grams of the prostate gland.

Gleason Score: A widely used method for classifying the cellular differentiation of cancerous tissue. The less the cancerous cells appear like normal cells, the more malignant the cancer. Two grades of 1-5, identifying the two most common degrees of differentiation present in the examined tissue sample, are added together to produce the Gleason score. High numbers indicate greater differentiation and more aggressive cancer. The grading system is named after its originator, Donald Gleason, M.D.

Globulin: Any of a number of simple proteins that occur widely in plant and animal tissues.

Gynecomastia: A side effect involving breast enlargement and tenderness, associated with various hormonal therapies that increase the level of estrogens in the body.

HDR Brachytherapy: High Dose Rate brachytherapy involves the temporary insertion of radioactive iridium isotopes into the prostate gland using transrectal ultrasound guidance.

Hematuria: Blood in the urine.

Hereditary: Inherited genetically from parents and earlier generations.

Holistic Medicine: Medical care, which considers the patient as a whole, including his or her physical, mental, emotional, spiritual, social and economic needs.

Hormone: A substance produced by one tissue or gland and transported by the bloodstream to another to effect or regulate physiological activity such as metabolism and growth.

Hormonal therapy: Cancer treatment involving the blockage of hormone production by surgical or chemical means. Because prostate cancer is usually dependent on male hormones to grow, hormonal therapy can be an effective means of alleviating symptoms and retarding the development of the disease.

Hormone Refractory PCa: Prostate cancer that is androgen independent, and therefore, unresponsive to hormonal therapies.

Hot Flash: A side effect of some forms of hormonal therapy, experienced as a sudden rush of warmth to the face, neck, and upper body.

Imaging: Radiology techniques that are often computer-enhanced and allow the physician to visualize areas inside the body that would not normally be visible.

Impotence: See Erectile Dysfunction.

Incontinence: A loss of urinary control. There are various kinds and degrees of incontinence. Overflow incontinence is a condition in which the bladder retains urine after voiding. As a consequence, the bladder remains full most of the time, resulting in involuntary seepage of urine from the bladder. Stress incontinence is the involuntary discharge of urine when there is increased pressure upon the bladder, as in coughing or straining to lift heavy objects. Total incontinence is the failure of ability to voluntarily exercise control over the sphincters of the bladder neck and urethra, resulting in total loss of retentive ability.

Inflammation: Redness or swelling caused by injury or infection.

Informed Consent: Permission to proceed given by a patient after being fully informed of the purposes and potential consequences of a medical procedure.

Intensity Modulated Radiation Therapy (IMRT): The most recent state-of-the-art, computer-aided technique for delivering higher doses of radiation more accurately than either conventional External Beam Radiation or Conformal Radiation.

Intermittent Androgen Deprivation (IAD): A temporary discontinuation of hormonal therapy that allows for a return to natural testosterone production in order to spare the patient from symptoms associated with androgen deprivation. Also referred to as Intermittent Hormonal Therapy (IHT).

Intravenous Pyelogram (IVP): A test that utilizes the injection of a special dye to check for the spread of cancer to the kidneys and bladder.

Investigational: A drug or procedure allowed by the FDA for use in clinical trials.

Isodose Line: A line or two-dimensional shape that circumscribes an area receiving a radiation dose greater than or equal to a specified amount.

Laparoscopic Lymphadenectomy: The removal of pelvic lymph nodes with a laparoscope via four small incisions in the lower abdomen.

LH (Luteinizing Hormone): A chemical signal originating in the pituitary gland that causes the testes to make testosterone.

LHRH Analogs (or LHRH Agonists): Synthetic compounds that are chemically similar to Luteinizing Hormone Releasing Hormone (LHRH), used to suppress testicular production of testosterone. The most commonly prescribed LHRH analogs are Lupron® and Zoldex®. See also Luteinizing Hormone-Releasing Hormone (LHRH).

LHRH Antagonist: A chemical agent that blocks the LHRH receptor without the testosterone surge associated with LHRH analogs. LHRH antagonists include Abarelix (Plenaxis®).

Linear Accelerator: A high energy x-ray machine generating radiation fields for external beam radiation therapy. These machines are typically mounted with a collimator (or multileaf collimator) in a gantry that rotates vertically around the patient being treated.

Localized Prostate Cancer: Cancer that is confined to the prostate gland, and therefore, considered curable.

Luteinizing Hormone-Releasing Hormone (LHRH): A chemical signal originating in the hypothalamus that causes the pituitary to make LH, which in turn stimulates the testicles to make testosterone.

Lymphadenectomy: The removal and examination of lymph nodes to precisely diagnose and stage cancer. See also Laparascopic Lymphadenectomy.

Lymph Node: A small, bean-shaped mass of tissue located throughout the body along the vessels of the lymphatic system. The lymph nodes filter out bacteria and other toxins, as well as cancer cells.

Magnetic Resonance Imaging (MRI): A painless, non-invasive technique using strong magnetic fields to produce detailed images of internal body structures. An MRI scan usually takes about 45 minutes.

Malignancy: A tumorous growth of cancer cells.

Malignant: Having the invasive and metastatic properties of cancer. Tending to become progressively worse and to result in death.

Margin: See Surgical Margin.

Metalloprotease Inhibitors: Drugs used to suppress the body's production of certain enzymes.

Metastasis: The spread of cancer, by way of the blood stream or lymphatic system, beyond the boundaries of the organ or structure where the cancer originated. Metastases is the plural. Metastatic refers to the characteristics associated with cancer that has spread or a secondary tumor.

Metastatic Work-Up: A group of tests, including bone scans, x-rays, and blood tests, to ascertain whether cancer has metastasized.

Monoclonal Antibody (mAb): An antibody that is directed against one specific protein (antigen).

Morbidity: Unhealthy consequences and complications resulting from treatment.

MRI: See Magnetic Resonance Imaging.

Nadir: The lowest point. Doctors sometimes use this as a verb to describe return of cancer or treatment failure. The PSA nadir refers to a minimum PSA value that should be maintained after treatment if the cancer has been successfully eradicated.

Necrosis: Death of cells or tissues caused by disease or injury.

Neoadjuvant: The use of a different type of therapy before primary, curative treatment. For example, neoadjuvant Androgen Deprivation Therapy is often used prior to radiation therapy or radical surgery, with the intent of improving the effectiveness of the primary treatment by reducing the size of the tumor and/or prostate gland.

Nerve-sparing: A procedure used during radical prostatectomy in which the surgeon attempts to save the nerves (neurovascular bundles) that allow for normal sexual functions.

Neurovascular Bundles: Strands of interwoven nerves and veins that run down the side of the prostate. The bundles contain microscopic nerves that are essential for erection; they also contain arteries and veins. Cutting the nerves in the bundles during surgery, or otherwise harming them in another procedure, usually renders the patient impotent.

Nocturia: Getting up at night to urinate.

Non-invasive: Not involving any incision in the body.

Oncogenes: Genes associated with tumor growth.

Oncology: The branch of medical science dealing with tumors. A medical oncologist is a specialist in the study of cancerous tumors.

Organ-confined Disease (OCD): Prostate cancer that is confined to the prostate capsule, as indicated clinically or pathologically.

Orchiectomy: A simple operation that involves surgical removal of the testicles, which produce most of the body's testosterone.

Osteoporosis: A decrease in bone mass and density causing fragility and porosity.

Overstaging: An assessment of an overly high clinical stage at initial diagnosis.

Palpable: Capable of being felt when examined by touch or manipulation.

PAP: See Prostatic Acid Phosphatase.

Pathologist: A doctor who specializes in the examination of cells and tissues removed from the body.

PBRT: See Proton Beam Radiation Therapy.

Perineum: The area of the body between the anus and scrotum. A perineal procedure uses this area as the point of entry into the body.

Perineural Invasion: Describing cancer, which has spread from the prostate to the perineum.

Periprostatic: Relating to the soft tissues immediately proximate to the prostate gland.

Photon: The quantum of electromagnetic energy, described as having zero mass and no electric charge. X-rays are high energy photons.

Placebo: A sugar pill often taken by participants in a medical study. Patients taking a placebo are compared to patients taking actual medications.

Ploidy Analysis: A pathological analysis to determine the number of sets of chromosomes in a cell.

Proctitis: Inflammation of the rectum.

Prognosis: A forecast of the course of a disease and future prospects of the patient.

Progression: A change in the status of the cancer indicating the condition has progressed and worsened.

Pro-oxidant: A term to describe substances that aid in oxidation.

Prostascint™ Scan: A method to determine whether or not cancer has spread to distant sites by using monoclonal antibodies. This test is especially helpful with patients who have been on hormonal therapy.

Prostate Capsule: The outer membranous covering of the prostate gland.

Prostatectomy: The surgical removal of part or all of the prostate gland.

Prostate Specific Antigen (PSA): A blood test that measures a substance manufactured solely by prostate gland cells. An elevated reading indicates an abnormal condition of the prostate gland, either benign or malignant. It is presently the most sensitive tumor marker for the identification and monitoring of prostate cancer.

Prostatic Acid Phosphatase (PAP): An enzyme produced by the prostate that is elevated (3.0 or higher) in many patients when prostate cancer has spread beyond the prostate.

Prostatitis: An infection or inflammation of the prostate gland that is treatable with medications.

Proton Beam Radiation Therapy (PBRT): A form of radiation therapy that utilizes protons as the source of energy (as opposed to X-rays or neutrons).

PSA: See Prostate Specific Antigen.

PSA Bounce (or PSA Bump): A rise in PSA level after first having a reduction in PSA after radiation therapy.

PSA Nadir: The lowest PSA value after a particular treatment.

PSA Velocity (PSAV): The rate of increase of the PSA level, expressed as nanograms per milliliter per year.

Radiation Therapy (RT): The use of high energy rays to kill cancer cells and malignant tissue.

Radiation Urethritis: Inflammation of the urethra caused by radiation therapy.

Radical Prostatectomy: An operation to remove the entire prostate gland and seminal vesicles.

Radiosensitivity: The degree to which a type of cancer responds to radiation therapy.

RBA or Relative Biological Effectiveness: A scale used to compare the intensity of radiation associated with various atomic particles.

Receptor: A cellular docking site that interacts with a specific protein or enzyme (called a ligand). The interaction typically leads to the synthesis of other substances such as proteins, hormones or enzymes.

Recurrence: Return of the cancer following remission or treatment intended as curative. Local recurrence indicates a return of the cancer at the site of origin. Distant recurrence indicates the appearance of one or more metastases of the disease.

Refractory: A term indicating that the cancer no longer responds to the current therapy.

Remission: Complete or partial disappearance of the signs and symptoms of the disease. The period during which a disease remains under control, without progressing. Even complete remission does not necessarily indicate cure.

Resection: The surgical removal of a part of an organ or structure.

Risk: The probability that a particular even will or will not happen.

RP: See Radical Prostatectomy.

RT: See Radiation Therapy.

Rx: The standard abbreviation for treatment.

Salvage Treatment: A medical tern for "Plan B." It means a patient must undergo another form of treatment because the first therapy was not successful. Salvage therapy does not always work and often has a greater degree of complications.

Saw Palmetto: A nutrient extracted from the saw palmetto shrub, which is considered by some to aid the body's immune system.

Seed Implantation (SI): A minimally invasive procedure by which radioactive seeds are implanted into the prostate gland to destroy cancer. Also referred to as seeding and brachytherapy.

Selenium: A non-metallic element thought to be beneficial as a nutrient; it is often included in multivitamin supplements.

Seminal Vesicles: Glands that, like the prostate, support male reproduction. Fluid secreted by these glands regulates the consistency of semen.

Side Effect: A reaction to a treatment or medication, usually referring to an undesirable effect.

Sphincter: A circular muscle which contracts to close an orifice. The urethral sphincter squeezes the urethra shut, providing urinary control.

Staging: The testing process by which the extent and severity of a known cancer is evaluated according to an established system of classification. It is used to help determine appropriate therapy. See TNM Staging and Whitmore-Jewett Staging.

Surgical Margin: The outer edge of the tissue removed during a radical prostatectomy. The surgical margin may be "negative," indicating that no cancer is present and a better prognosis, or "positive," indicating that not all of the cancer has been removed.

Systemic: Throughout the body and affecting the entire body.

T-Cell: An immune system cell or lymphocyte that directs an immune response to malignant or infected cells.

Testes: Two male reproductive glands located inside the scrotum. The testes are the primary sources for testosterone.

Testosterone: A male sex hormone chiefly produced by the testicles.

Thrombotic: Causing or relating to blood clotting.

TNM Staging: The most widely used classification system for evaluating the extent of prostate cancer. TNM refers to tumor, nodes and metastases. See Staging.

Transrectal: Through the rectum.

Transurethral: Through the urethra.

Transrectal Ultrasonography: See Ultrasound.

Transurethral Resection of the Prostate (TURP): A surgical procedure to remove tissue obstructing the urethra. The technique involves the insertion of an instrument called a resectoscope into the penile urethra, and is intended to relieve obstruction of urine flow due to enlargement of the prostate.

Tumor: An excessive growth of cells that is caused by uncontrolled and disorderly cell replacement. Abnormal tissue growth may be benign or malignant. See also Benign, Malignant.

TURP: See Transurethral Resection of the Prostate.

Ultrasound (Transrectal Ultrasonography): A painless, non-invasive diagnostic imaging technique using sound waves to create an echo pattern that reveals the structure of organs and tissues. It does not use x-rays.

Understaging: An overly low assessment of clinical stage at diagnosis.

Urethra: The tube that carries urine from the bladder and semen from the prostate out of the body through the penis.

Urologist: A physician who specializes in the diagnosis and the medical and surgical treatment of problems in the urinary and male reproductive systems.

Vasectomy: A surgical procedure to render a man sterile by cutting the vas deferens, thus eliminating the passage of sperm from the testes to the prostate.

Vasoactive: Causing the dilation or constriction of blood vessels.

Vesicle: A small sac containing fluid, as in seminal vesicles.

Whitmore-Jewett Staging: A classification system for evaluating the extent of prostate cancer. This system is less widely used for the designation of stage than is TNM staging.

X-rays: High energy radiation that can be used at low levels of intensity to make images of the body's internal structures, or at high intensity for radiation therapy.

QUESTIONS TO ASK YOUR DOCTOR

When first diagnosed with prostate cancer, a patient is likely to experience some degree of shock that may prevent him from absorbing the details of his case. Initially, the news of his condition may be all the patient can handle. But on a later visit, it is important for patients to obtain further information from the diagnosing physician. The checklist of questions below are intended to help the patient come to a better understanding of his condition, and to give him a foundation of knowledge for preparing to deal with his prostate cancer.

- ✔ How do you know I have prostate cancer?
- ✔ How far has the disease progressed?
- ✔ Before I decide on a course of treatment, what further tests should I have to determine the stage and nature of the cancer?
- ✔ What stage of prostate cancer do I have? How certain are you that my cancer is this stage?
- ✔ What are the treatment options for my stage of prostate cancer?
- ✔ Are there any treatment options other than those you have mentioned?
- ✔ What are the risks involved in each of the various treatments?
- ✔ What will happen if I am not treated?
- ✔ What treatment do you recommend, and why do you think it is best for me?

✔ Will the treatment that you recommend require hospitalization, or can it be performed on an out-patient basis?

✔ How many times have you performed this treatment in the last year?

✔ With the treatment you recommend, what is the rate and degree of impotence and incontinence among your patients?

✔ Does the site of the tumor in my prostate increase the risk of impotence or incontinence from the treatment you recommend?

✔ Is computerized planning sometimes involved in this treatment? Do you use such planning techniques? If not, why not?

✔ How will I feel during and after treatment?

✔ When will I be able to return to normal, everyday activities?

✔ When will I be able to resume sexual relations?

✔ What should I do if I experience erectile problems after treatment? Can you advise me or send me to someone who is an expert in the field?

✔ What should I do if I experience problems with incontinence after treatment? What can be done to treat incontinence? Is there an expert in the field you can refer me to in such an event?

✔ Will I need regular checkups to monitor the cancer and my response to treatment?

✔ What tests will be required for these check-ups, and what will they tell us?

✔ Are there particular warning signs for problems I should be aware of relating to a worsening of my condition or that might result from treatment?

✔ What do the different tests and treatments cost?

✔ How much of my medical expenses will my insurance cover and how much will I be required to pay out of pocket?

✔ Where should I go to get a second opinion?

Questions To Ask Your Doctor Regarding Prostate Brachytherapy

✔ Do you perform modern transperineal brachytherapy with either ultrasound or CT guidance (in contrast to open free hand retropubic implants of the 1970's)?

✔ Do you believe in modern transperineal brachytherapy or do you perform the procedure only because of an increase of demands placed upon you by your patients? (Patients are advised to avoid physicians who are offering seeding only to keep up with patient demand).

✔ How many modern brachytherapy procedures have you performed and for how many years?

✔ How did you learn the procedure? Have you had years of hands-on experience or did you start practicing more recently after a two to three day seminar? (Years of hands-on experience is obviously much preferable).

✔ Is there a regional center where I might find doctors who have a greater degree of experience doing modern implant brachytherapy than yourself?

✔ How do you ensure that the seeds have been correctly placed?

✔ Following the procedure (immediately, but also several weeks post-implant) will you be doing an analysis to determine if the seeds are properly placed?

✔ What do you do if the seeds are not properly positioned?

✔ I understand that many doctors' "successes and complications" are typically quoted from the major implant medical centers, but what are your success and complication rates? Have these been published in the medical literature?

✔ What are your rates of rectal injury? What are your rates of urinary incontinence? What is your rate of erectile dysfunction?

✔ What is your success rate with patients having my stage and/or grade of disease?

✔ Following the procedure, will you be the doctor who directly follows my progress?

✔ Could you provide me with the names of other patients who you have implanted (preferably years ago with similar stage, grade and age)?

✔ What role do you think hormonal therapy has in the treatment of prostate cancer with brachytherapy with regard to down-sizing and/or sensitization?

✔ What are your specific guidelines for performing implant therapy? Who do you consider candidates for the procedure?

✔ If appropriate: Are you aware of the fact that I have previously undergone a TURP? Is a TURP a contra-indication for brachytherapy performed by an experienced brachytherapist?

✔ If no doctors have much experience doing implants locally and if I'm not able to leave the area to be treated, might I consider undergoing a procedure with which you are more experienced? (Patients should note that an inexperienced brachytherapist, like an inexperienced surgeon, is of little value and should be avoided. There is no reason why you should be on the early end of your doctor's learning curve, whatever his specialty may be. If there are no experienced brachytherapists in your area, and if travel is not possible, then you may achieve better results with an experienced surgeon if one is available to you locally.)

✔ If I choose to be treated by a more experienced doctor (out of town, for example), will you continue to be my doctor at home without there being any hard feelings?

✔ What can I do if my cancer comes back after brachytherapy?

REFERENCES

Al-rimawi M. Griffiths DJ, Boake RC, Mador DR, Johnson MA. Transrectal ultrasound versus magnetic resonance imaging in the estimation of prostatic volume. Br J Urol. 1994 Nov;74 (5):596-600.

Badiozamani KR, Wallner K, Cavanagh W, Blasko J. Comparability of CT-based and TRUS-based prostate volumes. Int J Radiat Oncol Biol Phys. 1999 Jan 15; 43 (2):375-8.

Badiozamani KR, Wallner K, Sutlief S, Ellis W, Blasko J, Russell K. Anticipating prostatic volume changes due to prostate brachytherapy. Radiat Oncol Investig. 1999; 7 (6):360-4.

Banker RL. The preservation of potency after external beam irradiation for prostate cancer. Int J Radiat Oncol Biol Phys. 1988 Jul;15 (1):219-20.

Bartsch G, Egender G, Hubscher H, Rohr H. Sonometrics of the prostate. J Urol 1982; 127: 1119-1121.

Bates TS, Reynard JM, Peters TJ, Gingell JC. Determination of prostatic volume with transrectal ultrasound: A study of intra-observer and interobserver variation. J Urol. 1996 Apr;155 (4):1299-300.

Bazinet M, Karakiewicz PI, Aprikian AG, Trudel C, Peloquin F, Dessureault J, Goyal M, Begin LR, Elhilali MM. Reassessment of nonplanimetric transrectal ultrasound prostate volume estimates. Urology. 996 Jun; 47 (6):857-62.

Beyer D, Nath R, Butler, W, et al. American brachytherapy society recommendations for clinical implementation of NIST-1999 standards for (103)palladium brachytherapy. The clinical research committee of the American Brachytherapy Society. Int J Radiat Oncol Biol Phys. 2000 May 1;47(2):273-5.

Bice WS, Prestidge BR, Prete JJ, Dubois DF. Clinical impact of implementing the recommendations of AAPM Task Group 43 on permanent prostate brachytherapy using 125I. American Association of Physicists in Medicine. Int J Radiat Oncol Biol Phys. 1998 Mar 15; 40(5):1237-41.

Bice WS, Prestidge BR, Grimm PD, et al. Centralized multiinstitutional post-implant analysis for interstitial prostate brachytherapy. . Int J Rad Oncol Biol Phys. 1998; 41: 921-927.

Blasko JC, Grimm PD, Sylvester JE. Palladium-103 brachytherapy for prostate carcinoma. Int J Radiat Oncol Biol Phys. 2000; 46: 839-850.

Blasko JC, Mate T, Sylvester JE, Grimm PD, Cavanagh W. Brachytherapy for carcinoma of the prostate: techniques, patient selection, and clinical outcomes. Semin Radiat Oncol. 2002 Jan;12(1):81-94.

Chan TY, Partin AW, Walsh PC, et al. Prognostic significance of Gleason score 3+4 versus 4+3 tumor at radical prostatectomy. Urology. 2000; 56: 823-827.

Cheng S, Rifkin MD. Color Doppler imaging of the prostate: important adjunct to endorectal ultrasound of the prostate in the diagnosis of prostate cancer. Ultrasound Q. 2001 Sep; 17 (3):185-9.

Crook J, Esche B, Futter N. Effect of pelvic radiotherapy for prostate cancer on bowel, bladder, and sexual function: the patient's perspective. Urology. 1996 Mar; 47 (3):387-94.

Dattoli MJ, Sorace RA, Cash J, Wallner K. Biochemical failure rates following combination external beam radiation and Palladium-103 boost for clinically localized high risk prostate cancer: 10 year results. Int J Rad Oncol Biol Phys. 2002 Oct; 52 (2) (Supp.1): 38.

Dattoli MJ, Wallner K, A simple method to stabilize the prostate during transperineal prostate brachytherapy. Int J Rad Oncol Biol Phys. 1997; 38: 341-342.

Dattoli MJ, Wallner K, Sorace R, Ting J. Planned extracapsular seed placement using Palladium-103 for prostate brachytherapy. J. of Brachy Int. 2000; 16, 35-43.

Dattoli MJ, Wallner K, True L, Cash J, Sorace R. Long-term outcomes after treatment with external beam radiation therapy and palladium 103 for patients with higher risk prostate carcinoma: influence of prostatic acid phosphatase. Cancer 2003; 97:979-83.

Dattoli M, Wallner K, True L, Sorace R, Koval J, Cash J, Acosta R, Biswas M, Binder M, Sullivan B, Lastarria E, Kirwan N, Stein D. Prognostic role of serum prostatic acid phosphatase for 103Pd-based radiation for prostatic carcinoma. Int J Radiat Oncol Biol Phys. 1999 Nov 1; 45 (4):853-6.

Davis BJ, Haddock MG, Wilson TM, Rothenberg HJ, Bostwick DG, Herman MG, Pisansky TM. Treatment of extraprostatic cancer in clinically organ-confined prostate cancer by permanent interstitial brachytherapy: is extraprostatic seed placement necessary? Tech Urol. 2000 Jun; 6 (2):70-7.

Davis BJ, Pisansky TM, Wilson TM, Rothenberg HJ, et al. The radial distance of extracapsular extension of prostate carcinoma: implications for prostate brachytherapy. Cancer, 1999; 85: 2630-2637.

Dicker AP, Lin C-C, Leeper DB, Waterman FM. Isotope selection for permanent prostate implants? An evaluation of 103Pd versus 125I based on radiobiological effectiveness and dosimetry. Semin Urol Oncol. 2000 May; 18(2):152-9.

Feigenberg SJ, Wolk KL, Yang C-H, Morris CG, Zlotechi RA, Celecoxib to decrease urinary retention associated with prostate brachytherapy. Brachy 2 (June, 2003) 103-107.

Feldman HA, Goldstein I, Hatzichristou DG, et al. Impotence and its medical and psychosocial correlates: results of the Massachusetts Male Aging

Study. J Urol. 1994 Jan;151 (1):54-61.

Feleppa EJ, et al. Ultrasonic spectrum-analysis and neural-network classification as a basis for ultrasonic imaging to target brachytherapy of prostate cancer. Brachytherapy, 2002 (1) 48-53.

Forman JD, Kumar R, Haas G, Montie J. Neoadjuvant hormonal downsizing of localized carcinoma of the prostate: effects on the volume of normal tissue irradiation. Cancer Invest. 1995; 13 (1):8-15.

Gelblum DY, Potters L. Rectal complications associated with transperineal interstitial brachytherapy for prostate cancer. Int J Radiat Oncol Biol Phys. 2000 Aug 1; 48 (1):119-24.

Gelblum DY, Potters L, Ashley R, Waldbaum R, Wang X, Leibel S. Urinary morbidity following ultrasound-guided transperineal prostate seed implantation. Int J Rad Oncol Biol Phys. 1999; 45: 59-67.

Grimm PD, Blasko JC, Sylvester JE, Meier RM, Cavanagh W.10-year biochemical (prostate-specific antigen) control of prostate cancer with (125)I brachytherapy. Int J Radiat Oncol Biol Phys. 2001 Sep 1;51 (1):31-40.

Han B, Wallner K. Dosimetric and radiographic correlates to prostate brachytherapy-related rectal complications. Int J Cancer. 2001 Dec 20; 96 (6):372-8.

Han B, Wallner K, Aggarwal S, Armstrong J, Sutlief S. Treatment margins for prostate brachytherapy. Semin Urol Oncol. 2000 May; 18 (2):137-41.

Howard A, Wallner K, Han B, Schneider B, et al. Clinical course and dosimetry of rectal fistulas after prostate brachytherapy. J Brachy Int. 2001; (in press).

Hu L, Wallner K. Clinical course of rectal bleeding following I-125 prostate brachytherapy. Int J Radiat Oncol Biol Phys. 1998 May 1;41(2):263-5.

Hu L, Wallner K. Urinary incontinence in patients who have a TURP/TUIP following prostate brachytherapy. Int J Radiat Oncol Biol Phys. 1998 Mar 1; 40 (4):783-6.

Kagawa K, Lee WR, Schultheiss TE, Hunt MA, Shaer AH, Hanks GE. Initial clinical assessment of CT-MRI image fusion software in localization of the prostate for 3D conformal radiation therapy. Int J Radiat Oncol Biol Phys. 1997 May 1; 38 (2):319-25.

Khan MA, Partin AW. Management of high-risk populations with locally advanced prostate cancer. Oncologist. 2003;8(3):259-69.

Kim HL, Stoffel DS, Mhoon DA, Brandler CB. A positive caver map response poorly predicts recovery of potency after radical prostatectomy. Urology. 2000 Oct 1;56 (4):561-4.

Kleinberg L, Wallner K, Roy J, Zelefsky M, Arterbery VE, Fuks Z, Harrison L. Treatment-related symptoms during the first year following transperineal 125I prostate implantation. Int J Radiat Oncol Biol Phys. 1994 Mar 1; 28 (4):985-90.

Kollmeier MA, Stock RG, Stone NN. Urinary symptomatology and incontinence following post-brachytherapy transurethral resection of the prostate. Int J Radiat Oncol Biol Phys. 2003 Oct 1; 57 (2 Suppl):S439-40

Landis D, Wallner K, Locke J, Ellis W, Russell K, et al. Late urinary morbidity after prostate brachytherapy. (submitted 2002).

Lattanzi J, McNeely S, Hanlon A, Das I, Schultheiss TE, Hanks GE. Daily CT localization for correcting portal errors in the treatment of prostate cancer. Int J Rad Oncol Biol Phys. 1998; 41: 1079-1086.

Li Z, Palta JR, Fan JJ. Monte Carlo calculations and experimental measurements of dosimetry parameters of a new 103-Pd source. Med Phys 2000; 27: 1108-1112.

Ling CC. Permanent implants using Au-198, Pd-103 and I-125: radiobiological considerations based on the linear quadratic model. Int J Radiat Oncol Biol Phys. 1992; 23(1):81-7.

Ling CC, Li WX, Anderson LL, The relative biological effectiveness of I-125 and Pd-103. Int J Radiat Oncol Bio Phys, 1995; 32: 373-378.

Luse RW, Blasko J, Grimm P. A method for implementing the American Association of Physicists in Medicine Task Group-43 dosimetry recommendations for 125I transperineal prostate seed implants on commercial treatment planning systems. Int J Radiat Oncol Biol Phys. 1997 Feb 1;37 (3):737-41.

Maguire PD, Waterman FM, Dicker AP. Can the cost of permanent prostate implants be reduced? An argument for peripheral loading with higher strength seeds. Tech Urol. 2000 Jun; 6 (2):85-8.

Martinez A, Gonzalez J, Spencer W, Gustafson G, Kestin L, Kearney D, Vicini FA. Conformal high dose rate brachytherapy improves biochemical control and cause specific survival in patients with prostate cancer and poor prognostic factors. J Urol. 2003 Mar;169(3):974-9.

McNeal JE, Price HM, Redwine EA, Freiha FS, Stamey TA. Stage A versus stage B adenocarcinoma of the prostate: morphological comparison and biological significance. J Urol. 1988 Jan; 139 (1):61-5.

Meigooni AS, Sowards K, Soldano M. Dosimetric characteristics of the InterSource-103 palladium brachytherapy source. Med Phys 2000; 27: 1093-1100.

Merkle W. [Colour Doppler Transrectal 3D-Sonography of the Prostate–First Experiences]. Aktuel Urol. 2002 Jan; 33 (1):53-7. German.

Merrick GS, Butler WM. Modified uniform seed loading for prostate brachytherapy: rationale, design, and evaluation. Tech Urol. 2000 Jun; 6 (2):78-84. Review.

Merrick GS, Butler WM, Dorsey AT, Lief JH. Potential role of various dosimetric quality indicators in prostate brachytherapy. Int J Radiat Oncol Biol Phys. 1999; 44:717-724.

Merrick GS, Butler WM, Dorsey AT, Lief JH, Benson ML. Seed fixity in the prostate/periprostatic region following brachytherapy. Int J Rad Oncol Biol Phys. 2000; 46: 215-220.

Merrick GS, Butler WM, Dorsey AT, Lief JH, Totterd, Coram RJ. Influence of prophylactic dexamethasone on edema following prostate brachytherapy. Tech Urol. 2000 Jun;6(2):117-22. Int J Rad Oncol Biol Phys. 199; 43: 1021-1027.

Merrick GS, Butler WM, Dorsey AT, Lief JH, Walbert HL, Blatt HJ. Rectal dosimetric analysis following prostate brachytherapy. Int J Radiat Oncol Biol Phys. 1999 Mar 15; 43 (5):1021-7.

Merrick GS, Butler WM, Galbreath RW, et al. 5-year biochemical outcome following permanent interstitial brachytherapy for T1-T3 prostate cancer. Int J Radiat Oncol Biol Phys. 2001 Sep 1;51(1):41-8.

Merrick GS, Butler WM, Galbreath RW, Stipetich RL, Abel LJ, Lief JH. Erectile function after permanent prostate brachytherapy. Int J Radiat Oncol Biol Phys. 2002 Mar 15;52(4):893-902.

Merrick GS, Butler WM, Lief JH, Dorsey AT. Temporal resolution of urinary morbidity following prostate brachytherapy. Int J Radiat Oncol Biol Phys. 2000 Apr 1; 47 (1):121-8.

Merrick GS, Butler WM, Lief JH, Galbreath RW. Permanent Prostate Brachytherapy: Do Prostatectomy and External Beam Measure Up? J of Brachy Int., 2001 July-Sept, Vol. 17, 193.

Merrick GS, Butler WM, Lief JH, Stipetich RL, Abel LJ, Dorsey AT. Efficacy of sildenafil citrate in prostate brachytherapy patients with erectile dysfunction. Urology. 1999 Jun; 53 (6):1112-6.

Merrick GS, Butler WM, Tollenaar BG, Galbreath RW, Lief JH. The dosimetry of prostate brachytherapy-induced urethral strictures. Int J Radiat Oncol Biol Phys. 2002 Feb 1; 52 (2):461-8.

Merrick GS, Butler WM, Wallner KE, Galbreath RW, Lief JH. Long-term urinary quality of life after permanent prostate brachytherapy. Int J Radiat Oncol Biol Phys. 2003 Jun 1; 56 (2):454-61.

Merrick GS, Butler WM, Wallner KE, Lief JH, Anderson RL, Smeiles BJ, Galbreath RW, Benson ML.The importance of radiation doses to the penile bulb vs. crura in the development of postbrachytherapy erectile dysfunction. Int J Radiat Oncol Biol Phys. 2002 Nov 15 54 (4):1055-62.

Merrick GS, Wallner K, Butler WM. Management of sexual dysfunction after prostate brachytherapy. Oncology (Huntingt). 2003 Jan;17 (1):52-62; discussion 62, 67-70, 73.

Merritt CR. Doppler color flow imaging. J Clin Ultrasound. 1987 Nov-Dec; 15 (9):591-7.

Mizowaki T, Cohen GN, Fung AY, Zaider M. Towards integrating functional imaging in the treatment of prostate cancer with radiation: the registration of the MR spectroscopy imaging to ultrasound/CT images and its implementation in treatment planning. Int J Radiat Oncol Biol Phys. 2002 Dec 1; 54 (5):1558-64.

Nag S, Sweeney PJ, Wienthjes MG. Dose response study of Iodine-125 and Palladium-103 brachytherapy in a rat prostate tumor (Nb-Al-1). Endocur/ Hypertherm 1997; 9:97-104.

Narayana V, Roberson PL, Winfield RJ, Kessler ML. Optimal placement of radioisotopes for permanent prostate implants. Radiology. 1996 May; 199 (2): 457-60.

Narayana V, Roberson PL, Winfield RJ, McLaughlin PW. Impact of ultrasound and computed tomography prostate volume registration on evaluation of permanent prostate implants. Int J Radiat Oncol Biol Phys. 1997 Sep 1;39 (2):341-6.

Nathan MS, Seenivasagam K, Mei Q, Wickham JE, Miller RA. Transrectal ultrasonography: why are estimates of prostate volume and dimension so inaccurate? Br J Urol. 1996 Mar;77 (3):401-7.

Nath R, Anderson LL, Luxton G, et al. Dosimetry of interstitial brachytherapy sources: recommendations of the AAPM Radiation Therapy Committee Task Group No. 43. American Association of Physicists in Medicine. Med

Phys. 1995 Feb;22(2):209-34. Erratum in: Med Phys 1996 Sep;23(9):1579.

Nath R, Meigooni AS, Melillo A. Some treatment planning consideration for Pd-103 and I-125 permanent interstitial implants. Int J Radiat Oncol Biol Phys. 1992; 22: 1131-1138.

Peschel RE, Chen Z, Roberts K, Nath R. Long-term complications with prostate implants: iodine-125 vs. palladium-103. Radiat Oncol Investig. 1999;7(5):278-88.

Pierce LJ, Whittington R, Hanno PM, English W, Wein AJ, Goodman RL. Parmacologic erection with intracaverrnosal injection for men with sexual dysfunction following irradiation: a preliminary report. Int J Radiat Oncol Biol Phys. 1991 Oct; 21 (5):1311-4.

Pickett B, Fisch BM, Weinberg V, Roach M. Dose of radiation received by the bulb of the penis correlates with risk of impotence after three-dimensional conformal radiotherapy for prostate cancer. Urology. 2001 May;57(5):955-9.

Pound CR, Partin AW, Epstein JI, et al. Prostate-specific antigen after ana-tomic radical retropubic prostatectomy: patters of recurrence and cancer control. Urol Clin North Am. 1997; 24: 395-406.

Ragde H, Grado GL, Nadir BS. Brachytherapy for clinically localized pros-tate cancer: thirteen-year disease-free survival of 769 consecutive prostate cancer patients treated with permanent implants alone. Arch Esp Urol. 2001 Sep;54(7):739-47.

Rahmouni A, Yang A, Tempany C, Frenkel T. Accuracy of in-vivo assessment of prostate volumes by MRI and transrectal ultrasonography. J Comp Assist Tomo 1992; 16: 935-940.

Roach M, Faillace-akazawa P, Malfatti C, Holland J. Prostate volumes de-fined by magnetic resonance imaging and computerized tomographic scans for three-dimensional conformal radiotherapy. Int J Radiat Oncol Biol Phys. 1996 Jul 15; 35 (5):1011-8.

Roach M, Winter K, Michalski J, Bosch W, Lin X. Mean dose to the bulb of the penis correlates with risk of impotence at 24 months: preliminary analysis of Radiation Therapy Group (RTOG) phase I/II dose escalation trial 9406. Int J Radiat Oncol Biol Phys. 2000; 48: #2104.

Rosen MA, Goldstone L, Lapin S, Wheeler T, Scardino PT. Frequency and location of extracapsular extension and positive surgical margins in radical prostatectomy specimens. J Urol. 1992 Aug; 148 (2 Pt 1):331-7.

Roy AV, Brower ME, Hayden JE. Sodium Thymolphthalein monphosphate: a new acid phosphatase substrate with greater specificity for the prostatic enzyme in serum. Clin Chem. 1998; 17: 1093-1102.

Roy C, Buy X, Lang H, Saussine C, Jacqmin D. Contrast enhanced color Doppler endorectal sonography of prostate: efficiency for detecting peripheral zone tumors and role for biopsy procedure. J Urol. 2003 Jul; 170 (1):69-72.

Roy JN, Wallner K, Harrington PJ, Ling CC, Anderson LL. A CT-based evaluation method for permanent implants: Application to prostate. Int J Radiat Oncol Biol Phys. 1993; 26: 163-169.

Sauvain JL, Palascak P, Bourscheid D, Chabi C, Atassi A, Bremon JM, Palascak R. Value of power doppler and 3D vascular sonography as a method for diagnosis and staging of prostate cancer. Eur Urol. 2003 Jul; 44 (1):21-30; discussion 30-1.

Sethi A, Mohideen N, Leybovich L, Mulhall J. Role of IMRT in reducing penile doses in dose escalation for prostate cancer. Int J Radiat Oncol Biol Phys. 2003 Mar 15; 55 (4):970-8.

Shearer RJ, Davies JH, Gelister JS, Dearnaley DP. Hormonal cytoreduction and radiotherapy for carcinoma of the prostate. Br J Urol. 1992 May; 69 (5):521-4.

Sherertz T, Wallner K, Wang H, Sutlief S, Russell K. Long-term urinary function after transperineal brachytherapy for patients with large prostate glands. Int J Radiat Oncol Biol Phys. 2001 Dec 1;51(5):1241-5.

Shipley WU, Zietman AL, Hanks GE, Coen JJ, Caplan RJ, Won M, Zagars GK, Asbell SO. Treatment related sequelae following external beam radiation for prostate cancer: a review with an update in patients with stages T1 and T2 tumor. J Urol. 1994 Nov;152 (5 Pt 2):1799-805.

Sohayda C, Kepulian PA, Levin HS, Klein EA. Extent of extracapsular extension in localized prostate cancer. Urology. 2000 Mar; 55 (3):382-6.

Speight JL, Shinohara K, Pickett B, Weinberg VK, Hsu ICJ, Raoch M. Prostate volume change after radioactive seed implantation: possible benefit of improved dose volume histogram with perioperative steroid. Int J Radiat Oncol Biol Phys. 2000 Dec 1; 48 (5):1461-7.

Steinfeld AD, Donahue BR, Plaine L. Pulmonary embolizaiton of iodine-125 seeds following prostate implantation. Urol 1991; 37: 149-150.

Stock RG, Kao J, Stone NN. Penile erectile function after permanent radioactive seed implantation for treatment of prostate cancer. J Urol. 2001 Feb;165 (2):436-9.

Stock RG, Lo YC, Gaildon M, Stone NN. Does prostate brachytherapy treat the seminal vesicles? A dose-volume histogram analysis of seminal vesicles in patients undergoing combined PD-103 prostate implantation and external beam irradiation. Int J Radiat Oncol Biol Phys. 1999 Sep 1; 45 (2):385-9.

Stock RG, Stone NN, Kao J, Ianuzzi C, Unger P. The effect of disease and treatment-related factors on biopsy results after prostate brachytherapy. Cancer. 2000; 89:1829-1834.

Stock RG, Stone NN, Tabert A, Ianuzzi C, De Wyngaert JK. A dose-response study for I-125 implants. Int J Rad Oncol Biol Phys. 1998; 41: 101-108.

Stone RG, Ratnow ER, Stock NN. Prior transurethral resection does not increase morbidity following real-time ultrasound-guided prostate seed implantation. Tech Urol. 2000 Jun; 6 (2):123-7.

Stone NN, Stock RG. Prospective assessment of patient-reported long-term urinary morbidity and associated quality of life changes after 125-I prostate brachytherapy, J Brachy Int. 2003 March; 2 (1): 32-39.

Stone NN, Stock RG. Complications following permanent prostate brachytherapy. Eur Urol. 2002 Apr; 41 (4):427-33.

Sylvester JE, Blasko JC, Grimm PD, Meier R, Malmgren JA.Ten-year biochemical relapse-free survival after external beam radiation and brachytherapy for localized prostate cancer: the Seattle experience. Int J Radiat Oncol Biol Phys. 2003 Nov 15;57 (4):944-52.

Tapen EM, Blasko JC, Grimm PD, et al. Reduction of radioactive seed embolization to the lung following prostate brachytherapy. Int J Rad Oncol Biol Phys. 1998; 42: 1063-1067.

Teshima T, Hanks GE, Hanlon AL, Peter RS, Schultheiss TE. Rectal bleeding after conformal 3D treatment of prostate cancer: time to occurrence, response to treatment and duration of morbidity. Int J Radiat Oncol Biol Phys. 1997 Aug 1; 39 (1):77-83.

Tincher SA, Kim RY, Ezekiel MP, et al. Effects of pelvic rotation and needle angle on pubic arch interference during transperineal prostate implants. Int J Rad Oncol Biol Phys. 2000; 47: 361-363.

Wallner K, Blasko J, Dattoli MJ. Prostate Brachytherapy Made Complicated (Second Edition), Smart Medicine Press, Seattle, WA, 2001, p.4.6.

Wallner K, Lee H, Wasserman S, Dattoli M. Low risk of urinary incontinence following prostate brachytherapy in patients with a prior transurethral prostate resection. Int J Radiat Oncol Biol Phys. 1997 Feb 1; 37 (3):565-9.

Wallner K, Merrick G, True L, Cavanagh W, Simpson C, Butler W. I-125 versus Pd-103 for low-risk prostate cancer: morbidity outcomes from a prospective randomized multicenter trial. Cancer J. 2002 Jan-Feb;8(1):67-73.

Wallner K, Roy J, Harrison L. Dosimetry guidelines to minimize urethral and rectal morbidity following transperineal I-125 prostate brachytherapy.

Int J Radiat Oncol Biol Phys. 1995 May 15; 32 (2):465-71.

Wang H, Wallner K, Sutlief S, Blasko J, Russell K, Ellis W. Transperineal brachytherapy in patients with large prostate glands. Int J Cancer. 2000; 90: 199-205.

Waterman FM, Yue N, Corn BW, Dicker AP. Edema associated with I-125 or Pd-103 prostate brachytherapy and its impact on post-implant dosimetry: an analysis based on serial CT acquisition. Int J Radiat Oncol Biol Phys. 1998 Jul 15; 41 (5):1069-77.

Willins J, Wallner K. Time dependent changes in CT-based dosimetry of I-125 prostate brachytherapy. Radiat Oncol Invest 1998; 6:157-160.

Yu Y, Anderson LL, Li Z, Mellenberg DE, Nath R, Schell MC, Waterman FM, Wu A, Blasko JC. Permanent prostate seed implant brachytherapy: report of the American Association of Physicists in Medicine Task Group No. 64. Med Phys. 1999 Oct;26 (10):2054-76.

Zaider M, Zelefsky MJ, Lee EK, Zakian KL, Amols HI, Dyke J, Cohen G, Hu Y, Endi AK, Chui C, Koutcher JA. Treatment planning for prostate implants using magnetic-resonance spectroscopy imaging. Int J Radiat Oncol Biol Phys. 2000 Jul 1; 47 (4):1085-96.

Zelefsky MJ, Leibel SA, Burman CM, Kutcher GJ. Neoadjuvant hormonal therapy improves the therapeutic ratio in patients with bulky prostatic cancer treated with three-dimensional conformal radiation therapy. Int J Radiat Oncol Biol Phys. 1994 Jul 1; 29 (4):755-61.

Zelefsky MJ, McKee AB, Lee H, Leibel SA. Efficacy of oral sildenafil in patients with erectile dysfunction after radiotherapy for carcinoma of the prostate. Urology. 1999 Apr; 53 (4):775-8.

Zinreich, ES, Derogatis LR, Herpst J, Auvil G, Piantadosi S, Order SE. Pretreatment evaluation of sexual function in patients with adenocarcinoma of the prostate. Int J Radiat Oncol Biol Phys. 1990 Oct;19 (4):1001-4.

CHARTING YOUR PROGRESS

I t will be a great help to you to maintain a log of all tests and treatments you undergo during your battle with prostate cancer. This will accomplish several things. You will be able to supply on demand a history of your treatment to any physician you see. Following therapy, you will be able to personally keep an eye on your progress, and watch for any signs of recurrence. And rather than remain a mere bystander in your treatment program, you will be able to stay in charge of your own recovery.

The following pages include a Prostate Cancer Diagnostic Sheet, for recording the results of diagnostic tests, and a PSA Trend Chart, for visually charting changes in your PSA.

The Prostate Cancer Diagnostic Sheet lists the various diagnostic tests useful in the diagnosis and staging of prostate cancer. It is unlikely you will need to have all of these tests. However, proper diagnosis and staging will require that several of these tests be performed. Initial diagnosis is done with a digital rectal exam (DRE) and PSA blood test. If cancer is suspected, an ultrasound-guided biopsy should be performed.

Once cancer is detected, a battery of "staging" tests must be performed to determine the extent of the disease. The biopsy sample should be evaluated for differentiation and given a Gleason Score. The pathologist may also perform a DNA ploidy analysis. A bone scan is usually performed to check for spread of the cancer to the bones. Your doctor may also order a CT scan or MRI to visualize the extent and spread of cancer. Follow-up blood tests may include a second PSA test or a PAP blood test. In cases when the PSA is considerably elevated (over 20 ng/ml), a laparoscopic lymphadenectomy may be performed to see if cancer has invaded the lymph nodes. Before any test is performed, discuss its use and value in your case with your physician.

The PSA Trend Chart is an invaluable tool for the prostate cancer patient. For those engaged in "watchful waiting" to see if the disease progresses, the rate of rise in PSA values is a good indicator of the speed of disease progression. After treatment, a rising trend in PSA values probably signals treatment failure and recurrence of the disease. Be sure to discuss changes in your PSA, and the need for further tests or treatment, with your physician.

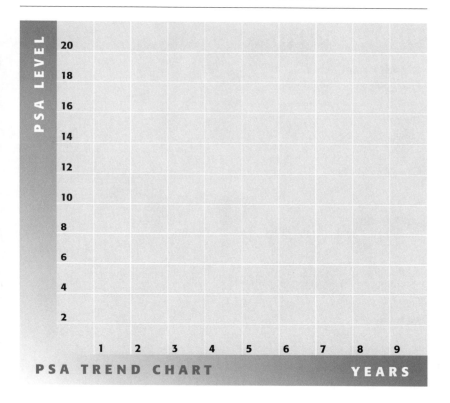

DIAGNOSTIC TEST	TEST RESULTS
Digital Rectal Exam (prostate size and shape)	
Biopsy (postive/negative)	
Gleason Score (value 2 to 10)	
DNA Ploidy (aneuploid, diploid, tetraploid)	
PSA Level (0 to greater than 1,000 ng/ml)	
PAP Level (0 to 100 ng/ml)	
Bone Scan (positive/negative)	
CT Scan (positive/negative lymph nodes)	
MRI (cancer confined to the prostate?)	
Ultrasound (cancer confined to the prostate?)	
Lymphadenectomy (positive/negative lymph nodes)	
Clinical Stage / Additional Notes	

NOTES

MY SUPPORT TEAM
Cancer Survivors, Doctors, Support Groups

Name: _____ Phone: _____

E-mail: _____

Name: _____ Phone: _____

E-mail: _____

Name: _____ Phone: _____

E-mail: _____

Name: _____ Phone: _____

E-mail: _____

Name: _____ Phone: _____

E-mail: _____

Name: _____ Phone: _____

E-mail: _____

Name: _____ Phone: _____

E-mail: _____

Name: _____ Phone: _____

E-mail: _____

Name: _____ Phone: _____

E-mail: _____

Name: _____ Phone: _____

E-mail: _____

Name: _____ Phone: _____

E-mail: _____

Name: _____ Phone: _____

E-mail: _____

Name: _____ Phone: _____

E-mail: _____

INDEX

U

V

W

X

Z

ABOUT THE AUTHORS

Michael J. Dattoli, MD

Michael J. Dattoli, MD, is a board-certified radiation oncologist with more than 15 years of brachytherapy experience and has performed thousands of prostate implant procedures. Dr. Dattoli has successfully applied the same technology to other forms of cancer, including breast, GI, GYN, sarcomas and lung malignancies. He is a noted author and speaker in this complex field of medicine. He received his Bachelor's degree in Science from Vassar College and completed his Medical Doctorate at Mount Sinai School of Medicine in New York City. He completed his resident training in Internal Medicine at Westchester County Medical Center and Affiliates in New York and his Radiation Oncology resident training at NYU Medical Center and Bellevue Hospital. Dr. Dattoli also served as chief fellow in Brachytherapy and Radiation Oncology at Memorial Sloan-Kettering Cancer Center in New York and at New York Hospital-Cornell University Medical Center prior to relocating to Florida.

Don Kaltenbach

Don Kaltenbach is the executive director of the Dattoli Cancer Center & Brachytherapy Research Institute. He is also a greater than 14-year prostate cancer brachytherapy survivor. He is a noted lecturer to men's groups across the country and has published award-winning books on the subject and a video recounting his journey to a cure via brachytherapy treatment. A former practicing attorney for nearly 30 years, Don has since dedicated his life's work to increasing awareness about prostate cancer. He is the founder of the Prostate Cancer Resource Network, a non-profit 501 (c)(3) tax-exempt organization created to educate and inform the public about prostate cancer and treatment options. The Network is sponsored by the Dattoli Cancer Foundation, which is devoted to research efforts for improved treatment of prostate cancer, educational seminars and expanded public awareness.

Jennifer C. Cash, MS, ARNP, OCN®

Jennifer C. Cash, MS, ARNP, OCN is an Advanced Registered Nurse Practitioner, Certified Oncology Nurse, Clinical Nurse Specialist and an integral part of the Dattoli Cancer Center Team. She is widely recognized for her particular expertise in all aspects of brachytherapy. Ms. Cash has an extensive background in Medical Surgical Oncology, Radiation Oncology and brachytherapy. She received her Bachelor's of Science degree and Master's of Science degree in nursing from the University of South Florida. She is a noted author and speaker on the subjects of brachytherapy, sophisticated radiation delivery systems (3DCRT and IMRT), and hormonal therapies.

OUR MISSION

Seneca House Press is sponsored by the Dattoli Cancer Foundation, a 501(c)(3), tax-exempt charitable organization, whose mission is

- ✔ to raise awareness of the wide-spread incidence of Prostate Cancer and the need for early and annual screenings;
- ✔ to provide information and support to men newly diagnosed with Prostate Cancer, and
- ✔ to foster research into better diagnostic tools and treatment options for Prostate Cancer.

Visit our Web site at: http://www.dattolifoundation.org

TO ORDER

To order additional copies of SURVIVING PROSTATE CANCER WITHOUT SURGERY, please write or call:

Seneca House Press/Dattoli Cancer Foundation
PO Box 50773
Sarasota, FL 34232-0306

Please enclose $18.95 U.S. (25.95 Canada) plus $3.95 shipping and handling. Checks should be made payable to the Dattoli Cancer Foundation.

To order by credit card:

Individual orders: (800) 580-6866

Quantity Orders: (800) 915-1001

By Fax: (941) 330-2317

ALSO AVAILABLE FROM
SENECA HOUSE PRESS

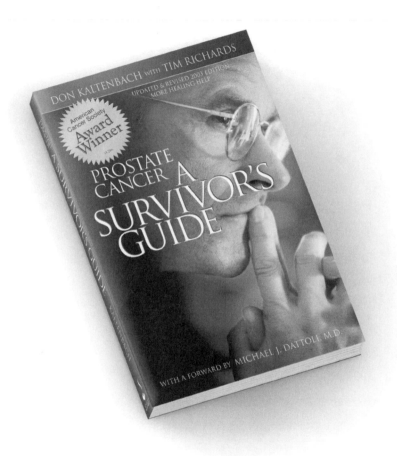

One man's emotional journey from diagnosis to recovery.
No one understands like someone who has been through it.

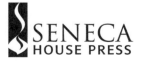

THE WARNING SIGNS OF PROSTATE CANCER

There are often no warning signs of prostate cancer. However, in some cases the following may indicate the presence of the disease:

- ✔ Elevated or rising PSA
- ✔ Abnormal Digital Rectal Exam
- ✔ Blood in urine
- ✔ Pain or difficulty urinating
- ✔ Increased urge to urtinate, especially at night
- ✔ Hesitant or intermittent urinary flow
- ✔ Pain or discomfort in area of prostate
- ✔ Unusual and unexplained weight loss
- ✔ Continual pain in lower back, hips or pelvis